DIABETIC DIET AFTER 50 COOKBOOK

Precise And Easy Recipes To Manage Diabetes With A Low-carb And Low-sugar Diet. Includes Colorful Images And A 30-day Meal Plan.

Freddy Quincy

© Copyright 2024 by Freddy Quincy - All rights reserved.

The content of this book is provided with the intent to offer accurate and reliable information. However, by purchasing this book, you acknowledge that neither the publisher nor the author claim expertise in the topics discussed, and any advice or recommendations are provided solely for entertainment purposes. It is recommended that you consult with professionals as necessary before taking any action based on the content of this book.

This disclaimer is recognized as fair and valid by both the American Bar Association and the Committee of Publishers Association, and is legally binding across the United States.

Unauthorized transmission, duplication, or reproduction of any part of this work, whether electronic or printed, including the creation of secondary or tertiary copies, or recorded versions, is prohibited without the express written consent of the publisher. All rights not expressly granted are reserved.

The information presented in this book is deemed to be truthful and accurate. However, any negligence in the use or misuse of this information by the reader is their sole responsibility, and under no circumstances will the publisher or the author be liable for any consequences or damages that may arise from the use of this information.

Furthermore, the information contained in this book is intended solely for informational purposes and should be treated as such. No guarantees are made regarding the ongoing validity or quality of the information. Trademarks mentioned are used without permission and their inclusion does not constitute an endorsement by the trademark holder.

TABLE OF CONTENTS

- **INTRODUCTION** 7
- **UNDERSTANDING DIABETES AFTER 50** 9
- **HOW TO MANAGE DIABETES** 15
- **MACRONUTRIENTS AND MICRONUTRIENTS** 23
- **FOODS TO EMBRACE AND FOODS TO AVOID** 29
  - **Foods to Embrace for Diabetics Over 50:** 35
  - **Foods to Avoid for Diabetics Over 50:** 37
- **BREAKFAST** 39
  - Broccoli and Feta Omelet 39
  - Chia and Almond Yogurt Parfait 40
  - Spinach and Mushroom Egg Muffins 40
  - Chia and Hemp Seed Yogurt Parfait 40
  - Turmeric Tofu Scramble 41
  - Smoked Salmon and Avocado Tartine 41
  - Berry Ginger Zinger Smoothie 42
  - Cucumber Melon Medley Shake 42
  - Peaches and Cream Oat Shake 42
  - Chia and Coconut Yogurt Parfait 43
  - Savory Muffin Tin Omelettes 43
  - Smoked Salmon and Herb Cream Cheese Wraps 44
- **LUNCH** 45
  - Seared Tuna and Avocado Salad 45
  - Beetroot and Goat Cheese Arugula Salad 46
  - Cucumber and Fennel Citrus Salad 46
  - Broccoli and Cheddar Soup 47
  - Tomato Basil Soup 47
  - Tempeh and Kale Pesto Wrap 48
  - Spicy Pumpkin Soup 48
  - Quinoa & Black Bean Salad Jars 49
  - Smoked Chicken Caesar Lettuce Wrap 49
  - Sardine and Chickpea Salad Pita 50
  - Chicken and Walnut Pesto Wraps 50
  - Mediterranean Tuna and Barley Salad 50
- **DINNER** 53
  - Zucchini Ribbon and Turkey Bacon Skillet 53
  - Lemon Herb Roasted Chicken Thighs 54
  - Grilled Tofu and Asparagus with Tahini Sauce 54
  - Spiced Cauliflower Steaks with Turmeric and Cumin 55
  - Zesty Lemon Garlic Tilapia 55
  - Cauliflower Steaks with Romesco Sauce 56
  - Zucchini Ribbon Salad with Lemon and Herbs 56
  - Slow-Cooked Mediterranean Chicken 57
  - Stuffed Bell Peppers with Quinoa and Turkey 57
  - Herb Crusted Salmon with Fennel Salad 58

 Tuscan Pork Tenderloin 58
 One-Pan Salmon with Asparagus 59

SNACKS AND SIDES 61

 Roasted Chickpea and Kale Poppers 61
 Zucchini Basil Bites 62
 Roasted Red Pepper and Walnut Dip 62
 Cucumber Roll-Ups with Feta and Sun-dried Tomatoes 63
 Herbed Ricotta and Chive Spread 63
 Spicy Pumpkin Seed Dip 63
 Spicy Bok Choy in Garlic Sauce 64
 Roasted Acorn Squash with Herbs and Pecans 64
 Cauliflower Tabbouleh 65
 Rosemary-Spiced Nuts 65
 Chilled Cucumber Cups 66
 Smoked Salmon & Cream Cheese Pinwheels 66

DIABETIC-FRIENDLY DESSERTS 67

 Almond Flour Lemon Bars 67
 Coconut Chia Pudding 68
 Almond Flour Lemon Cake 68
 Almond Butter Chocolate Energy Balls 69
 Spiced Baked Pear Halves 69
 Pumpkin Spice Muffins with Stevia 70
 Coconut Flour Chocolate Chip Cookies 70
 Grilled Peach with Ricotta and Basil 71
 No-Bake Lemon Cheesecake Cups 71
 Strawberry Rhubarb Compote with Mint 72
 Pistachio and Date Bars 72
 Blueberry Mango Chia Pudding 72

30 DAYS MEAL PLAN 74
CONCLUSION 77
MEASUREMENT CONVERSION TABLE 79

INTRODUCTION

Welcome to your new adventure in culinary wellness. If you've picked up this book, chances are you're eager to transform your diet into one that manages your blood sugar levels, enriches your health, and aligns with your lifestyle as you strive for longevity and well-being. It's both an exciting and a daunting journey, and I'm here to guide you every step of the way.

Turning fifty is a milestone marked by rich experiences and, often, the need to pay closer attention to our health. This period of our lives can bring new challenges, among them managing diabetes or pre-diabetic conditions. The good news? You are capable of embracing this challenge and thriving beyond it. This cookbook is tailored specifically to ease the burden of finding diabetic-friendly recipes that are as nourishing as they are delicious.

Throughout the pages, you will discover not just recipes, but gateways to a healthier you. I've carefully crafted each dish to ensure it respects your dietary needs without compromising on flavor or satisfaction. Forget the bland and uninspiring meals you might fear come with a diabetes diagnosis; think instead of vibrant plates brimming with nutrients that invite your senses to a feast.

What sets this cookbook apart is its commitment to simplicity and empowerment. I understand the constraints and the demands of daily life—especially for those not accustomed to cooking regularly. Each recipe is designed to be straightforward, quick, and using ingredients readily available at your local supermarket. Furthermore, we'll walk through meal planning for a full 30 days, easing you into this new way of eating without feeling overwhelmed.

As we progress, remember it's not just about following recipes—it's about rewriting your health story. You may encounter frustrations or setbacks, such as dietary limitations at social events or the fear of diabetes-related complications. Rest assured, such concerns are tackled here, turning each challenge into an opportunity for success.

With this book as your companion, you're not just cooking; you're cultivating a lifestyle that makes room for more health and more joy—well after 50.

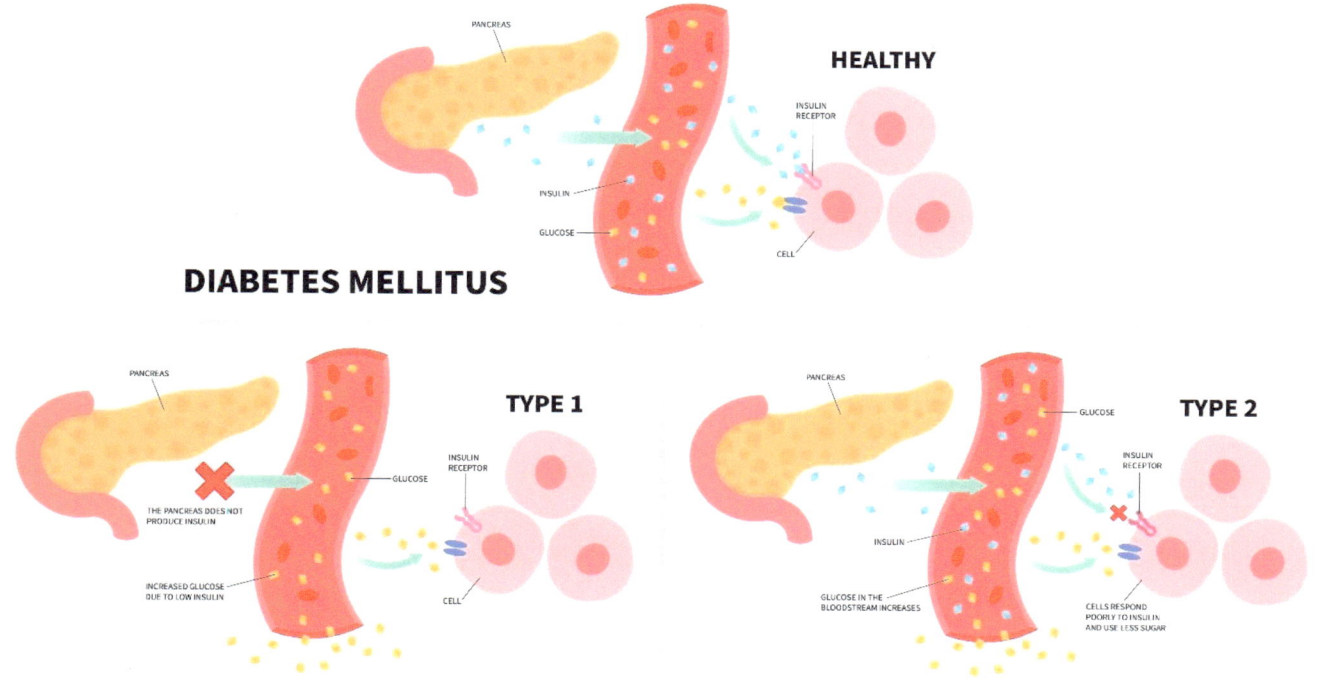

Understanding Diabetes After 50

Navigating life post-50 can be an invigorating chapter of discovery and reinvention, but for many, it also brings the unwelcome debut of health complications such as type 2 diabetes. This disease silently weaves its way into lives, often spurred on by decades of unchecked habits and the natural toll of aging on our bodies. Understanding diabetes in this light is not just about recognizing its symptoms and medical implications—it's about accepting and adapting to a lifestyle that can control and, quite possibly, improve the quality of your life.

When you cross the threshold into your fifties, your body begins to tell stories of the past: maybe a knee that stiffens up from an old injury or a back that reminds you of years of hard work. For some, glucose levels in their blood begin to narrate a new tale, one where the metabolism isn't as forgiving with sugars and carbohydrates as it once was. This is a crucial juncture where knowledge can transform into power—the power to manage, mitigate, and meet the challenges of diabetes head-on.

In this chapter, we delve into what it means to live with diabetes after 50. It's not merely about adhering to a new set of dietary rules or mourning the loss of certain foods but embracing a full, vibrant life that considers dietary choices as tools for wellness, not restrictions. We'll explore how the body changes with age and how these changes impact blood sugar management. From the pancreas' diminishing insulin production to the liver's glucose regulation, every organ has a part in this complex dance of hormones and health.

Beyond physiological insights, this chapter aims to equip you with an understanding that empowers resilience in the face of diabetes. We'll discuss how to navigate social meals, holiday feasts, and solitary snacks with equal aplomb, maintaining blood sugar levels without losing the joy of eating. Discover how every meal becomes an opportunity to support your body's needs, crafting a life not defined by diabetes, but informed by it.

The Science of Diabetes: How It Affects the Body After 50

Imagine a finely tuned orchestra, each instrument contributing to a harmonious performance. This symphony is akin to how our body functioned in our younger years. As we age, particularly crossing the milestone of 50, this orchestra begins to play a slightly different tune, especially regarding how our bodies process glucose, leading to an increased risk of diabetes.

Diabetes, primarily type 2, emerges from a complex interplay between genetic factors and lifestyle choices. However, its prevalence in those over 50 sheds light on how aging itself changes our bodily functions. Let's explore the science behind diabetes and why these changes are more pronounced as we age.

As we step into the later decades of life, our pancreatic function alters. The pancreas, responsible for producing insulin — the hormone that regulates blood sugar levels — starts to tire. Its insulin-producing cells, the beta cells, lose their efficiency. This decline is not abrupt but rather a gradual descent, which means the early signs can often go unnoticed. Simultaneously, our body's cells become less responsive to insulin, a condition known as insulin resistance. Initially, the pancreas compensates by working harder and producing more insulin, but over time, this compensatory mechanism wears out. Imagine trying to unlock a door with a key that doesn't fit quite right. No matter how much you jiggle the key (or how much insulin is present), the lock (cells needing glucose for energy) doesn't budge easily.

The problem extends beyond just the pancreas and cell receptors. Our liver, which plays a pivotal role in storing and releasing glucose, also undergoes changes. Normally, the liver balances glucose release and storage precisely, but with insulin resistance, this balance is disrupted, often leading to higher glucose levels in the blood, particularly problematic after fasting or between meals.

Further complicating matters is the accumulation of visceral fat — fat stored within the abdominal cavity — common in aging adults. This type of fat is not merely an inert storage of excess calories but an active player in hormonal and inflammatory processes that contribute to insulin resistance.

Apart from these physical transformations, aging impacts glucose metabolism through changes in muscle mass. Muscles are voracious glucose consumers. As we age, we naturally lose muscle mass, a condition known as sarcopenia. With less muscle mass, our body's capacity to utilize glucose diminishes, again contributing to higher blood sugar levels.

These biological shifts are compounded by lifestyle factors that often accompany aging. Physical activity tends to decrease, dietary patterns may waver, and cumulative stress over the years can take its toll, influencing everything from hormone function to sleep patterns and mood, all of which play roles in metabolic health.

Against this backdrop of physiological changes, managing diabetes requires a nuanced approach. It's not merely about reducing sugar intake but understanding and adapting to how your body now behaves. Monitoring blood glucose levels becomes crucial. It's not just about avoiding sweets; it's about understanding the glycemic impact of all foods and how different types of exercise can affect your glucose levels.

Moreover, managing diabetes after 50 isn't just a physical challenge but a psychological one as well. The mental load of managing a chronic condition, along with the normal stresses of aging, can affect your mental well-being. Acknowledging and addressing these psychological factors is as important as managing the diet.

Finally, another layer to this complex condition is the varied response to medication. Medications that might have worked when you were younger might not be as effective or might come with different side effects as your body changes. This necessitates a closer collaboration with healthcare providers to tailor a management plan that is as unique as your personal physiological makeup.

Diabetes after 50 presents a distinct set of challenges, steeped in the broader narrative of aging. Yet, understanding these changes not only demystifies the condition but also empowers you to take proactive steps. Managing diabetes effectively at this stage of life integrates a holistic understanding of body, mind, and lifestyle, ensuring that the melody of life, though different, plays on beautifully and harmoniously. Herein lies the power to not just survive with diabetes but thrive despite it, embracing the golden years with vigor and vitality.

Common Symptoms and Early Detection

In the journey of life after 50, our bodies often whisper secrets about our health through symptoms that can initially seem as benign and inconspicuous as a gentle breeze on a quiet day. Oftentimes, these whispers are the early signs of diabetes, which, if heard early, can significantly alter the management and progression of the disease. Recognizing these subtle changes is akin to understanding a new language, one that can save lives and improve the quality of living for those affected.

Diabetes, largely silent in its initial stages, tends to announce its presence through a series of indicators that can easily be mistaken for normal signs of aging. Frequent urination, for instance, can often be brushed off as a mere consequence of getting older. However, it's essential to understand that this symptom arises from the body's struggle to regulate and manage high blood sugar levels, compelling the kidneys to work overtime to filter and absorb the excess glucose.

Thirst follows suit, not just a thirst that a glass of water can quench but a persistent, nagging kind of thirst. This isn't the body crying out for water because of a hot day or because you've just finished a long walk. This type of thirst is the body's response to a high concentration of glucose in the blood, pulling fluid from tissues, leaving you more dehydrated than the norm.

Another herald of diabetes is increased hunger, even when you are eating adequately. This happens because diabetes prevents your cells from accessing glucose for energy due to insulin resistance or the lack of insulin production, sending signals to your brain that you need to eat more.

Weight loss, particularly unexpected and unexplained, is another red flag. Despite eating more, you might find the scales tipping in the opposite direction. This weight loss isn't the result of fat reduction but rather the loss of water weight and muscle mass, as the body burns fat and muscle for energy, unable to utilize glucose properly.

Fatigue in diabetes is a compound problem. Not only is the body unable to use glucose for energy efficiently, but high blood sugar levels can also lead to inflammation, further draining your energy. It feels more profound than just needing an extra cup of coffee; it's a kind of tiredness that rests in your bones, unshaken by sleep or rest.

Vision changes often catch many by surprise. High blood sugar levels can cause the lens of the eye to swell, changing your ability to see. These vision changes can fluctuate, sometimes clear and at other times blurred, depending on blood sugar levels. It might be tempting to attribute this to old age, but it's a sign that needs a closer look, literally and figuratively.

Less discussed but equally important are the symptoms that involve sensation, such as tingling or numbness in the hands and feet. This condition, known as neuropathy, arises when excess glucose damages nerve fibers. It's a change that can easily be set aside as a consequence of sleeping awkwardly or mere pins and needles, but it's one of the body's more dire ways of signaling a deeper problem.

Recognizing these symptoms early can be like catching a smoldering fire before it flames. It provides an opportunity to manage and potentially reverse diabetes or prevent its most severe complications. Early detection means routine checks, being attuned to the changes in your body, and having honest conversations with your healthcare provider about any changes, no matter how small they may seem.

Screening tests play a pivotal role in early detection. Simple blood tests such as the A1C, which doesn't require fasting, can provide insights into your average blood sugar levels over the last two to three months. Other tests include fasting blood sugar tests and oral glucose tolerance tests. These are not just for those who exhibit symptoms but are recommended as routine screenings for individuals over the age of 45. Understanding these symptoms and taking proactive steps towards detection can not only curb the advancement of diabetes but also pave the way for a healthier life post-50. It's about listening to the body's whispering secrets and responding with measures that enhance quality and vitality of life. With the right knowledge and actions, you can continue to dance through life's stages with grace and strength, proving that while diabetes can be a fact of life, it doesn't need to define your life.

Risk Factors and Causes of Diabetes in Older Adults

As the golden years unfold, the risk of developing diabetes looms larger, influenced by a tapestry woven from diverse threads that encompass lifestyle, genetic predisposition, and unforeseen changes in the body's regulatory mechanisms. Understanding the myriad factors that escalate the risk of diabetes in older adults isn't just a matter of medical insight but a crucial strategy for prevention and early intervention.

Firstly, aging itself is a non-negotiable risk factor that we all eventually face. As we age, the body's systems gradually lose efficiency, and this includes the pancreas's ability to produce insulin, as well as the cells' ability to respond to it effectively. However, age is just the backdrop against which other risk factors may come into play.

Genetics also plays a significant role. Just like inheriting your father's knack for storytelling or your mother's eye color, the blueprint for diabetes can also be passed down through generations. If your family history includes parents or siblings with diabetes, your own risk significantly escalates. Even with a healthy lifestyle, genetics can tilt the balance, making vigilance and regular screenings essential.

Our weight, particularly as we move deeper into middle age and beyond, tends to find new, stubborn places to settle, predominantly around the abdomen. This visceral fat is not merely a nuisance regarding wardrobe choices—it also functions differently from the fat elsewhere in our bodies. It is metabolically active, increasing insulin resistance, and propagating inflammatory processes that further risk diabetes.

A sedentary lifestyle magnifies the risk. Physical activity does far more than burn calories; it helps regulate blood sugar levels, boosts sensitivity to insulin, and contributes to maintaining a healthy weight. The less active you are, the greater the risk of diabetes becomes, as the body fails to utilize glucose efficiently.

Dietary patterns play an equally pivotal role. A diet high in refined sugars and saturated fats but low in fiber can contribute to weight gain and affect insulin sensitivity, directly influencing diabetes development. Conversely, a diet rich in whole grains, fruits, vegetables, and lean proteins can help mitigate this risk.

Ethnicity is another facet that cannot be overlooked. Certain ethnic groups, such as African Americans, Hispanic Americans, Native Americans, and some Asian Americans, are at a higher risk of developing diabetes. This increased risk is a complex interplay of genetics, diet, socioeconomic status, and health behaviors that differ across various communities.

Furthermore, the presence of other health conditions such as hypertension and high cholesterol is intricately linked with diabetes. Often bundled together as metabolic syndrome, these conditions each heighten the risk of developing diabetes and suggest an overall pattern of declining metabolic health.

Sleep patterns also influence diabetes risk. Quality sleep is not just about quantity but also about the rhythm and timing. Disrupted sleep patterns or conditions like sleep apnea can affect how your body uses insulin, raising blood sugar levels and possibly leading to diabetes over time.

Polycystic Ovary Syndrome (PCOS) is specifically relevant for women entering their post-reproductive years. While PCOS can start in the reproductive years, its effects can extend far beyond, with insulin resistance as a key component of the syndrome, setting the stage for the development of diabetes later in life.

Stress, both physical and emotional, should not be underestimated as a contributor to diabetes. Chronic stress affects the body in myriad ways, one being the release of stress hormones, which can raise blood sugar levels. Beyond biological stress, psychological stress related to changes in lifestyle, financial stress, or loss of loved ones, which can be more prevalent in older age, also impacts metabolic health.

Finally, previous cases of gestational diabetes or prediabetes are potent indicators of an increased risk. These conditions suggest that the body has already shown signs of struggling with glucose regulation, signaling the need for monitoring and preemptive lifestyle changes.

Armed with knowledge about these risk factors, individuals are better positioned to engage in preventive measures or, if necessary, early interventions that can significantly alter the trajectory of their health journey post-50. This awareness isn't just about guarding against diabetes but embracing a lifestyle that enhances overall vitality and wellness in the later chapters of life. With each risk factor identified and addressed, the narrative of life after 50 can be rewritten, emphasizing health, activity, and preventive care.

Long-Term Health Implications and Complications

Navigating the terrain of diabetes after ages 50 may suddenly feel like carrying a little extra weight, not just physically, but emotionally and mentally as well. The consequences of diabetes blooming at this stage of life often extend beyond the immediate blood sugar management issues. They grow roots deep into various aspects of health, potentially bringing a bouquet of complications if left unchecked.

The impact on the cardiovascular system is one of the most significant and dangerous repercussions of unmanaged diabetes. High blood sugar levels can lead to the build-up of deposits in the arteries, increasing the risk of atherosclerosis. Atherosclerosis can then lead to life-threatening heart conditions such as heart attacks and strokes. This link underscores why heart checks are not just about monitoring cholesterol and blood pressure but also about keeping a close eye on glucose levels.

Kidney health is also at stake. The kidneys, responsible for filtering waste from the blood, can become overwhelmed by the excess glucose running through your system. Over time, this strain can lead to diabetic nephropathy, a severe form of kidney disease, which often slowly creeps up, showing minimal symptoms until it reached advanced stages. This complication is a prime example of why regular kidney function tests are vital for those diagnosed with diabetes.

One of the more visibly disturbing complications might involve the eyes, a condition known as diabetic retinopathy. High glucose levels damage the tiny blood vessels in the retina, potentially leading to blurred vision and, in severe cases, blindness. The eyes may be the windows to the soul, but in the context of diabetes, they are also indicators of how well diabetes is being managed.

Neuropathy, or nerve damage, is a common fallout of diabetes that can result in numbness, tingling, or even pain, usually in the hands or feet. This not only affects quality of life but also increases the risk of injury, as wounds might not be felt and thus not promptly treated. Neuropathy is insidious, starting as a mild inconvenience and potentially leading to more severe complications such as amputations if infections occur and are left unmanaged.

The skin, the largest organ of the body, also doesn't escape the effects of diabetes. High sugar levels can lead to dry, itchy skin and make skin infections more likely. These skin issues are not merely cosmetic; they are signals that the diabetes may not be under optimal control.

Mental health is another critical aspect affected by diabetes. Managing a chronic condition can strain mental fortitude, leading to bouts of depression or anxiety. The worry about maintaining proper blood sugar levels, the stress of dietary restrictions, and the fear of potential complications can take a considerable toll on one's mental health.

Joint and mobility issues might also emerge as diabetes progresses. High glucose levels can affect the musculoskeletal system, leading to conditions like frozen shoulder or carpal tunnel syndrome, which interfere significantly with daily activities and quality of life.

Moreover, those with diabetes are more susceptible to infections due to an impaired immune system. From more common infections like the flu to more severe conditions such as pneumonia, the body's reduced ability to heal itself can turn what would normally be minor health issues into serious complications.

Addressing these long-term implications isn't just about fear management; it's about proactive engagement with your health. Regular consultations with healthcare professionals, routine monitoring of your blood sugar levels, effective management plans tailored to individual needs, and lifestyle adjustments are paramount.

In essence, the journey doesn't end at managing sugar levels but extends into a more holistic approach towards health that considers not just the physical but also the psychological aspects of living with diabetes. Armed with knowledge and the right tools, managing diabetes effectively can transform the twilight years from a period of worry and discomfort to one of health and enjoyment.

How to Manage Diabetes

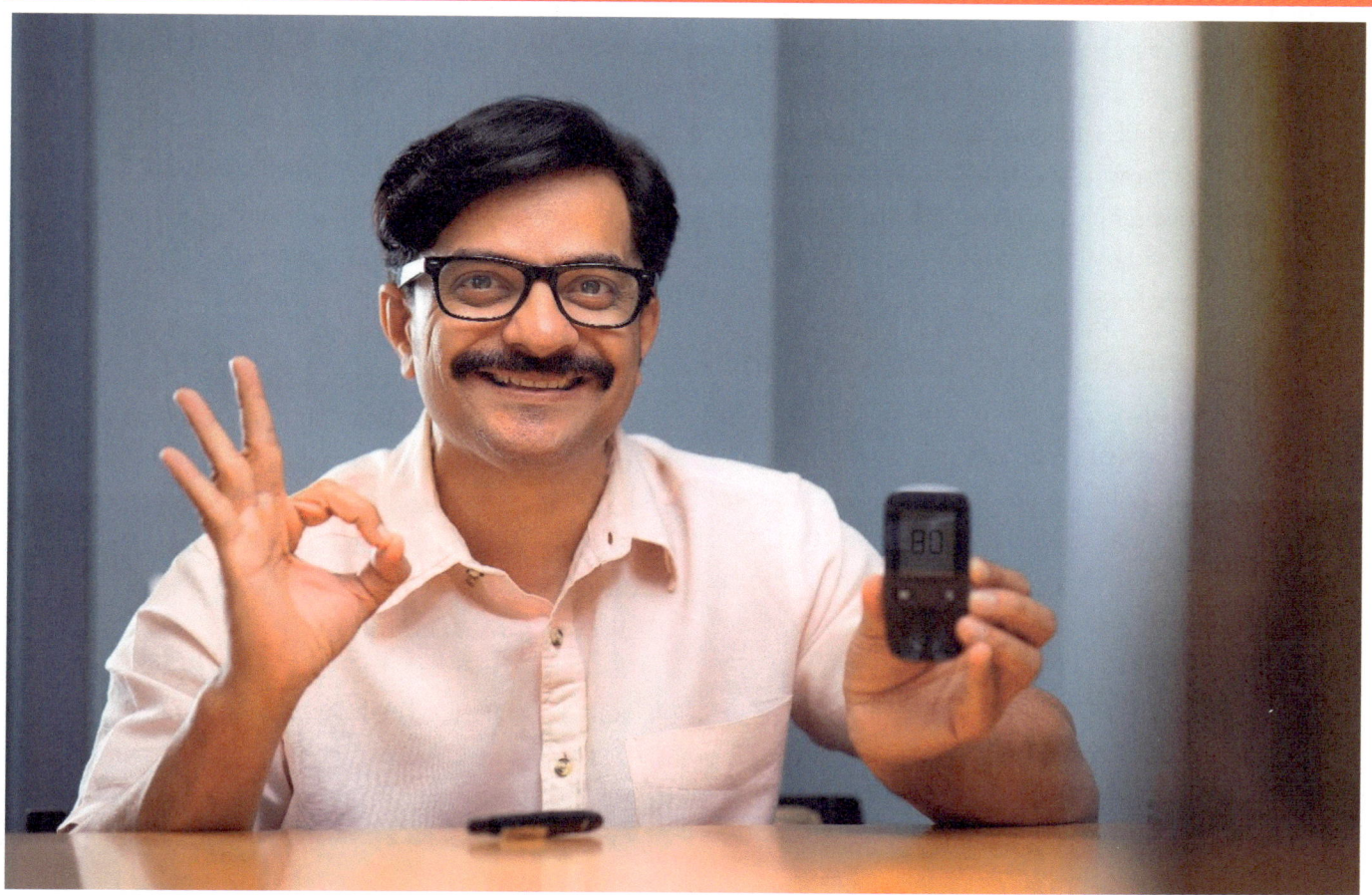

Managing diabetes, especially after the age of 50, often feels like navigating a maze with constantly shifting walls. New dietary needs, changing physical health, and the psychological burden of managing a chronic condition can make each day feel unpredictably challenging. Yet, amidst these complexities, there lies a powerful tool—your diet—which, when managed correctly, can significantly stabilize and improve your diabetic condition.

Picture this: you wake up feeling in control, not because your diabetes has magically disappeared, but because you have harnessed the knowledge of what to eat and how it affects your body. In this chapter, you will learn precisely that. We will delve into understanding the relationship between food and blood sugar levels. Think of your diet as a calming balm, a way to gently steer your glucose levels into a safe and healthy range.

The key to success here is knowing that no single magical diet suits everyone. Instead, think about tailoring your nutritional intake based on what your body responds to best. We'll explore how to incorporate low-carb and low-sugar foods in a way that doesn't make mealtimes a scientific experiment but rather an enjoyable, stress-free experience. Remember, the goal is to enjoy your food while keeping those numbers on the glucose meter in check. Beyond the types of food, portion control is your hidden ally. It's not just about avoiding sugar but understanding how much to eat and when. The joy of eating can still be yours, but with a new perspective on how much is enough.

Lastly, we will tackle the inevitable curveballs—those social gatherings, holiday feasts, and eating out—that can make sticking to a diabetic-friendly diet seem daunting. Here, you'll gain strategies not just to survive but to thrive in these situations without feeling isolated or deprived.

By the end of this chapter, the hope is not just that you'll know more about managing diabetes but that you'll feel equipped and confident to make choices that support a vibrant, healthful life despite diabetes. Here's to embracing each meal as an opportunity for nurturing your body and enriching your life.

Monitoring Blood Sugar Levels: Tools and Techniques

Imagine having a compass that guides you through the dense forest of diabetes management; that compass is your ability to monitor blood sugar levels effectively. Understanding and utilizing this tool effectively can turn what often seems like a thorny path into a manageable journey. Whether you're just beginning to navigate this path or you've been trekking through it for years, the tools and techniques of monitoring your blood sugar levels can redefine your daily life by giving you control and confidence.

Monitoring your blood sugar is not merely about keeping track of numbers. It's about interpreting what those numbers mean in the context of your day-to-day life. Everyday activities like eating, physical activities, and even stress have significant impacts on your blood sugar levels. By tracking these levels, you create a detailed map of how your body responds to different situations, empowering you to make healthier choices and avoid potential complications.

The Significance of Regular Monitoring

Regular blood sugar monitoring is a cornerstone of managing diabetes. Think of your body as a business, and the blood glucose monitor as your accountant, recording every transaction. Just as a good business needs to know where it stands financially, a well-maintained body needs to know its glucose levels. This regular checking can tell you if your body is 'running in the red', allowing you to take immediate corrective measures.

Choosing the Right Tools

There are several tools at your disposal for monitoring glucose levels, each with its own set of advantages. Traditional blood glucose meters are like reliable old friends, straightforward and familiar. They work by analyzing a small drop of your blood, typically drawn from your fingertip, to give you a glucose reading within seconds.

In recent years, continuous glucose monitors (CGMs) have risen in popularity. These devices provide a more high-tech solution, giving you real-time, dynamic glucose readings throughout the day and night. A sensor inserted under the skin typically on the abdomen or arm, measures glucose levels in tissue fluid. It offers a constant stream of data to your smartphone or dedicated device, plotting your glucose level in a graph that illustrates your body's ups and downs. This continuous feedback loops in a more comprehensive picture, letting you adjust quickly and efficiently.

Perfecting the Technique

No matter which tool you choose, the key to obtaining accurate readings largely depends on your technique. Ensure cleanliness by washing your hands before taking a sample. Let your hands dry completely as any residual water can dilute your blood sample, leading to inaccuracies. When using a traditional meter, rotate your testing sites between fingers and occasionally use the side of your fingertip, which is less sensitive.

Calibration is also critical, especially for CGMs. The process may vary between devices, but it generally involves confirming the accuracy of the CGM with a traditional blood glucose meter and adjusting as necessary. This ensures that the readings you get are both accurate and reliable.

Interpreting the Numbers

Understanding what these numbers mean is vital in managing your diabetes effectively. Blood sugar levels are typically measured in milligrams per deciliter (mg/dL) or millimoles per liter (mmol/L), depending on geographical location. Generally, a reading between 70 to 130 mg/dL before meals and less than 180 mg/dL two hours after starting a meal is considered within target for most people with diabetes, but your targets may differ based on your specific circumstances and health status.

More than simply aiming for 'good' numbers, consider the patterns and trends over days and weeks. Are your morning numbers steadily rising? Does a specific type of meal tend to spike your sugar levels? These insights can guide necessary adjustments in your diet and lifestyle.

Managing the Emotional Side of Monitoring

Frequent monitoring can sometimes lead to frustration. A high reading can make you feel like you've failed, whereas a good reading can provide an undue sense of security. It's important to approach your results with a mindset of curiosity rather than judgment. Each reading is a data point, a clue to how well your management plan is working or an indicator that it's time to adjust your strategy.

Remember, these tools are not here to judge but to empower you. They are part of a larger narrative of your health and wellness journey, helping you to tune in more closely to your body's needs. Managing diabetes is as much about understanding the significance of these numbers as it is about learning what to do about them.

Moving Forward With Confidence

As you continue to monitor your blood sugar, think of each day as an opportunity to learn more about your diabetes and take control. With the right tools and techniques, along with an understanding of what the numbers mean, you can maintain not just a healthy body, but a vibrant, fulfilling life even with diabetes.

Embracing these methods is not just about keeping complications at bay; it's about enhancing your quality of life, allowing you more freedom and peace of mind. Diabetes, after all, is a manageable condition, and with precise and consistent monitoring, you're equipped to live life on your terms.

The Role of Medication and Insulin Management

As we navigate the journey of managing diabetes, especially later in life, medication and insulin often become integral parts of the daily routine. Understanding how these tools fit into your diabetes management strategy can significantly influence your quality of life, offering you a sense of empowerment and control over your condition.

Medication and insulin management might initially seem daunting—almost like learning a new language or adjusting to driving in a foreign country. However, with proper guidance and a clear understanding, they morph from daunting to doable, turning into reliable allies in your diabetes management.

Understanding Diabetes Medication

Medications for managing diabetes are not one-size-fits-all. They work in various ways to help reduce blood sugar levels, improve insulin sensitivity, and sometimes aid in weight management, which can be a significant aspect of diabetes care after 50. The most commonly prescribed medications fall into several categories, each with a specific role in managing blood sugar levels effectively:

- **Sulfonylureas** stimulate your pancreas to produce more insulin.
- **Metformin** enhances your body's sensitivity to insulin and helps reduce the amount of glucose your liver releases.
- **DPP-4 inhibitors** help to increase insulin production and decrease glucose production.
- **GLP-1 receptor agonists** slow digestion and help lower blood sugar levels.

The choice of medication, or combination thereof, depends largely on individual factors including your specific type of diabetes, your blood sugar levels, any other health conditions, and how your body responds to each medication.

The Critical Role of Insulin

Insulin therapy can sometimes be perceived with undue apprehension. Yet, it's one of the most effective methods to manage glucose levels in the body. For many people with Type 2 diabetes, especially those diagnosed later in life, insulin becomes a necessary addition to their treatment plan as their condition progresses.

Insulin isn't just one substance; it comes in various forms designed to work at different speeds and durations. These include:

- **Rapid-acting insulin**, which starts working within a few minutes and is effective for a short period, is typically taken before meals.
- **Long-acting insulin** covers insulin needs for about one full day and is usually administered at night.
- **Premixed insulin**, a combination of specific proportions of immediate and extended-release insulin, simplifying dosing but requiring strict adherence to schedule.

Integrating insulin into your life doesn't mean loss of independence or flexibility; rather, it signifies a commitment to managing your diabetes effectively. Insulin pens, pumps, and new continuous glucose monitoring systems have made administering insulin less invasive and more manageable.

Perfecting Your Technique and Timing

The effectiveness of both oral medications and insulin depends not just on 'what' and 'how much', but on 'when' and 'how' they are taken. It's crucial to take your medication at the same time each day to maintain steady blood sugar levels. For insulin, techniques such as rotating the injection sites and proper storage of insulin ensure that each dose is as effective as possible. The nuances of timing your insulin with meals, snacks, and physical activities are essential skills that need honing over time with practice and patience.

Addressing Fears and Misconceptions

Common misconceptions around insulin, like the fear of injections or beliefs about insulin causing health decline, need addressing. Insulin therapy, when managed well, can dramatically improve your life quality. It's not a sign that your diabetes has worsened, but rather a step towards better health management.

The Emotional and Psychological Aspects

Beyond the physical management of medication and insulin, there's an emotional terrain to navigate. It's common to experience feelings of frustration or sadness about needing medication or insulin. However, viewing these treatments as tools for maintaining your health can help shift your perspective from resistance to acceptance and proactive management.

Managing medications and insulin requires not just understanding what they do, but also integrating them into your daily life, which includes emotional adaptation. Joining support groups, either online or in person, can be beneficial. Sharing experiences and tips with peers who understand what you're going through can be incredibly supportive and enlightening.

Continuing Education and Consultation

Staying informed through continual learning and regular consultations with your healthcare provider is vital. Treatment paradigms in diabetes care are constantly evolving, and keeping abreast with these changes can help you make the most informed decisions about your health care.

Conclusion

In essence, embracing the role of medication and insulin in managing your diabetes is akin to learning how to balance a bicycle. Once you master the balance, the path forward becomes smoother and the journey less daunting. Medications and insulin aren't just necessities; they are part of a holistic approach to a healthier, more vibrant life despite diabetes. With the right knowledge and support, you can turn these tools into assets, fostering better health management and a more joyous journey through life.

Incorporating Exercise: Physical Activity for Diabetes Control

In managing diabetes, especially after 50, incorporating exercise into your daily routine is akin to cultivating a garden; it requires patience, persistence, and a touch of passion. But once the seeds of habit are planted and nurtured, the health benefits grow exponentially, offering more than just improved blood sugar control—they can enliven your entire well-being.

Embracing Activity: The Why and the How

The benefits of physical activity for anyone, especially those managing diabetes, are immense. Exercise helps increase insulin sensitivity, meaning your body will use available insulin more effectively. It also aids in regulating blood glucose levels, not to mention promoting heart health, reducing stress, and increasing overall energy levels. For individuals past the age of 50, these benefits also include enhanced mobility and improved muscle mass, which naturally decline with aging.

Yet, the idea of incorporating a new exercise routine can sometimes feel daunting. You might ponder, "How can I begin?" or "What if I haven't been very active?" The key is starting with gentle, achievable steps.

Finding the Right Fit: Tailoring Your Exercise Regimen

The first step is to consult with your healthcare provider to ensure any new exercise plan accommodates your health needs. Next, consider activities you enjoy—whether it's gardening, walking through your neighborhood, swimming, or even light cycling. The enjoyment factor is crucial; it transforms exercise from a chore into a cherished part of your day.

Building Slowly: From Little Acorns Grow Mighty Oaks

For those new to regular physical activity, or returning after a long hiatus, starting slowly is paramount. A gradual increment in activity level helps your body adjust without overwhelming it. You might start with a ten-minute walk each day, gradually increasing the duration and intensity as your fitness improves. The aim is not to run marathons (unless that excites you!) but to weave more movement into your daily life in a pleasurable and sustainable way.

Monitoring Impact: Exercise and Blood Sugar Levels

One of the most empowering aspects of exercise for those with diabetes is the tangible impact it has on blood sugar levels. Monitoring your levels before and after exercise can provide motivating feedback and also ensure your safety. Noticing how different activities influence your glucose can help you fine-tune your routine for maximum benefit.

It's also wise to be prepared for how your body responds to exercise. Keep a small, healthy snack or glucose tablet with you in case your blood sugar drops too low, particularly if you are on insulin or certain diabetes medications.

Overcoming Challenges: Physical Limitations and Safety Measures

If physical limitations constrain you, adaptations can ensure you still reap the benefits of exercise. Chair exercises, water aerobics, and light resistance band workouts can provide less strain on the joints while still enhancing muscle strength and flexibility. The key is to focus on what you can do and find ways to adapt movements to your ability level.

Safety is also paramount. Wear proper footwear, stay hydrated, choose safe environments for your activities, and always warm up and cool down to prevent injuries. Listen to your body's signals—pushing through pain is not advisable, particularly when managing a condition such as diabetes.

Social and Mental Wellbeing: The Broader Benefits of Activity

Beyond the physical health improvements, exercise also plays a crucial role in social and mental wellbeing. Joining a walking group or taking a class at a local community center can not only make activities more enjoyable but also connect you with others, combating loneliness and keeping your spirits high.

Furthermore, regular physical activity is known to significantly boost mood and reduce anxiety and depression through the release of endorphins, often referred to as the body's natural 'feel-good' hormones. For many managing diabetes, this emotional lift can be just as valuable as the physical benefits.

Embedding Exercise into Everyday Life

Make physical activity a natural part of your daily routine. Perhaps you could walk while catching up with a friend over the phone, take the stairs instead of the elevator, or engage in light stretching while watching television. These habits, once integrated into your life, help maintain blood sugar control and enhance your overall health without seeming like a burden.

In Closing: The Lifelong Journey

Incorporating exercise into your diabetes management plan isn't just about immediate benefits; it's an investment in your future health. Creating and maintaining an active lifestyle can ensure you not only manage your diabetes more effectively but also improve your quality of life, providing you with years of activity, independence, and well-being.

Remember, the journey of a thousand miles begins with a single step. Start where you are, use what you have, and do what you can. Over time, these small steps will lead to significant changes, crafting a healthier, more energetic you, capable of living life fully and joyfully, even with diabetes.

Stress and Sleep: How They Impact Blood Sugar Management

In the labyrinth of managing diabetes, particularly in later years, two often overlooked factors play crucial roles in your blood sugar levels: stress and sleep. Like invisible threads, they weave through your daily life, significantly impacting your diabetes management and overall well-being.

The Silent Disruptors: Stress and Its Implications on Diabetes

Stress, a common companion in our fast-paced world, is not merely a mental or emotional inconvenience. It has tangible physical effects, particularly on blood glucose levels. When you experience stress, your body prepares to "fight or flight" by releasing hormones such as adrenaline and cortisol. These hormones raise your blood sugar by making the body more resistant to insulin. For someone managing diabetes, this reaction can complicate blood sugar control extensively.

Furthermore, chronic stress not only disrupts your glucose levels but can also lead to poor dietary choices, reduced physical activity, and a neglect of regular blood sugar monitoring. Acknowledging the impact of stress is the first step in mitigating its effects. Techniques such as deep breathing exercises, yoga, and mindfulness meditation have been found to effectively reduce stress and, in turn, help manage blood sugar levels more effectively.

Crafting Calm: Practical Strategies for Stress Management

Creating a personal toolbox for stress management can transform your approach to handling diabetes. It could include activities that you find calming and enjoyable, such as reading, gardening, or listening to music. Regular engagement in these activities can provide a counterbalance to stress, acting as a buffer that shields your body from the harsh impacts of stress hormones.

Integrating stress management techniques into your daily routine—like starting your day with a meditation session or ending it with a gratitude journal—can significantly alleviate stress. This proactive approach not only keeps your blood sugar levels steadier but also enhances your overall quality of life.

The Power of Sleep: More Than Just Rest

Sleep and diabetes management are intricately linked. A good night's sleep does more than just recharge your body; it helps regulate the hormones that control appetite and insulin regulation. Lack of sleep can lead to higher levels of cortisol, which increases blood sugar levels, and can make you more insulin resistant. Adults typically need between 7 to 9 hours of quality sleep per night. However, many individuals with diabetes experience disturbances in their sleep patterns, whether due to symptoms of high blood sugar like frequent urination or from worries that spike cortisol levels through the night.

Sleep Strategies for Better Diabetes Management

Improving sleep quality and duration can directly influence your diabetes control. Establishing a calming bedtime routine—such as avoiding caffeine and heavy meals before bed, minimizing exposure to blue light from screens, and creating a comfortable, dark sleep environment—can enhance your sleep quality.

If sleep apnea, a common condition among those with diabetes, is part of the problem, treating it can markedly improve your sleep quality and thus your diabetes management. Consultations with a healthcare provider to discuss sleep problems can uncover underlying issues like sleep apnea, which are manageable with the right interventions.

Synchronized Systems: How Stress and Sleep Interact

The relationship between stress and sleep forms a cycle; poor sleep can increase stress levels, while high stress can lead to poor sleep quality. Recognizing this cycle is crucial as breaking it can have a significant positive impact on managing your diabetes. Engaging in physical activities can be an excellent method to combat both stress and sleep issues. Exercise releases endorphins, natural mood lifters, and promotes better sleep by physically tiring out the body.

Tailoring Your Approach: Individual Needs and Responses

Each individual's experience with stress and sleep is unique, especially when managing a condition like diabetes. It's essential to monitor how changes in stress and sleep affect your blood sugar readings and adjust your management strategies accordingly. Keeping a diary of stress levels, sleep hours and quality, along with daily blood sugar levels, can provide clear insights into how these variables interact.

In Conclusion: Integrating Knowledge into Life

Recognizing the profound impact of stress and sleep on diabetes management allows for more effective control and an improved quality of life. By addressing these areas thoughtfully and persistently, you set the stage not just for better health metrics but for a more fulfilling, energetic life.

As you move forward, remember that managing these aspects of your life is not just about better diabetes control; it's about crafting a life that is rich, enjoyable, and healthy. The journey with diabetes is not just about the food you eat or the medicine you take, but about how you live each day, how well you rest each night, and how effectively you melt away the stress that life invariably brings.

MACRONUTRIENTS AND MICRONUTRIENTS

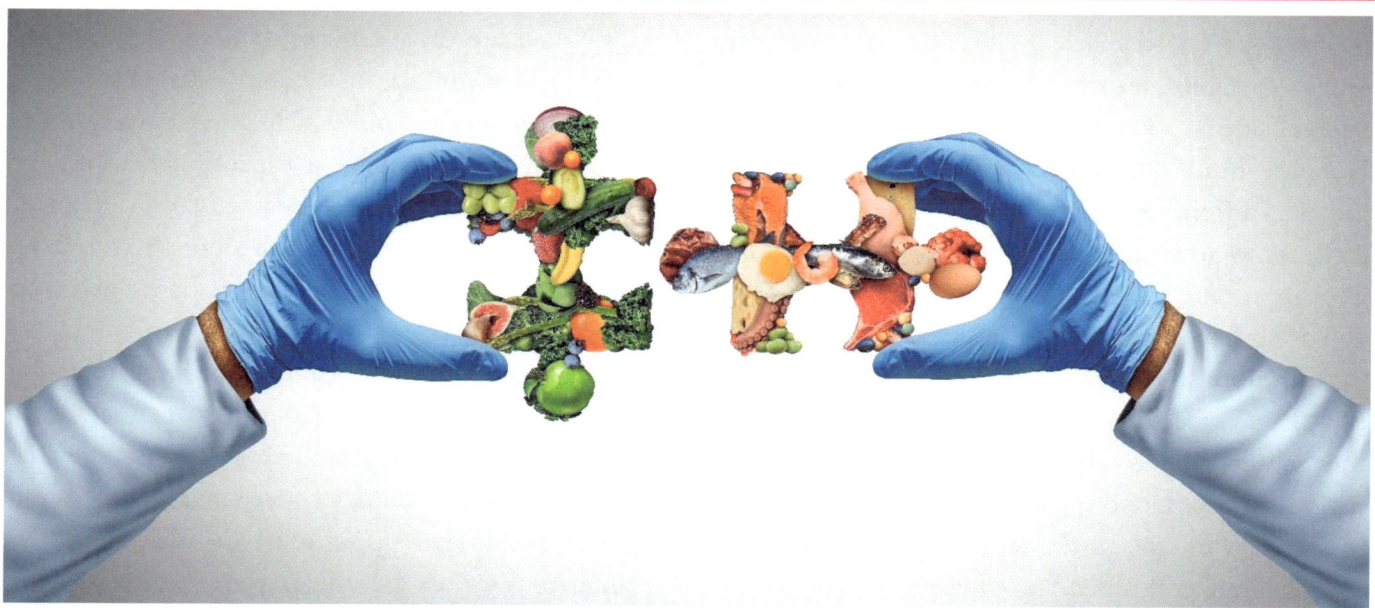

Navigating the landscape of a diabetic-friendly diet after 50 can sometimes feel a bit like being a scientist in your kitchen — measuring, calculating, and experimenting with various combinations of foods. But at the heart of each meal preparation lies the robust backbone of all nutrition — macronutrients and micronutrients.

Macronutrients, which include carbohydrates, proteins, and fats, are often spotlighted in the context of diabetes management because of their direct impact on blood sugar levels. However, understanding their role isn't just about limitation; it's about making informed choices. For instance, opting for complex carbohydrates like leafy greens and whole grains can provide the glucose control needed without the rapid spikes associated with refined sugars. Similarly, the right kinds of fats and proteins can not only satiate but also aid in long-term energy regulation and cellular repair.

Micronutrients, though required in smaller amounts, play no less critical roles. Vitamins and minerals from a spectrum of colorful vegetables and fruits — think deep greens, vibrant reds, and rich yellows — contribute not just to the visual appeal of your plate but to your overall health. They help fight inflammation, bolster your immune system, and repair cellular damage, which is crucial in managing diabetes complications.

As we peel back the layers of dietary advice peppered through this book, understanding macronutrients and micronutrients offers you more than just scientific insight; it provides the keys to a more empowered approach to your diabetic diet. Each recipe in this cookbook strives not only to meet your dietary needs but to enrich your body with the necessary tools for a robust, vibrant life. So, as we explore these essential nutrients, imagine yourself mastering the delicate balance of flavors and nutritional content, crafting meals that delight both the palate and the body. Through knowledge and practical application, take joy in each meal as a step towards managing your diabetes with confidence and ease.

Understanding Carbohydrates and Their Impact on Blood Sugar

Carbohydrates have often been cast as the villains in the story of diabetes management. But understanding the nuanced role of carbohydrates and their impact on blood sugar levels can transform them from foes to allies, guiding us toward better health and more enjoyable meals.

When we talk about carbohydrates, we're referring to a diverse group of foods, from the sugar in your morning coffee to the complex fibers in your leafy green vegetables. It's a broad category, encompassing simple sugars such as glucose and fructose, and complex forms like starch and dietary fiber. Each interacts differently with your body, particularly when it comes to how they affect your blood sugar levels.

To appreciate these differences, let's start by exploring how carbohydrates influence glucose levels in your bloodstream. When you consume carbs, your body breaks them down into simpler sugars which are then absorbed into the bloodstream. This process typically causes blood sugar levels to rise. The rate and magnitude of this rise depend on the type of carbohydrate consumed.

Simple carbohydrates, often found in sugary snacks and processed foods, are quickly digested, leading to a rapid spike in blood sugar. This can be particularly troubling for individuals managing diabetes, as their bodies struggle to regulate these sudden highs. Conversely, complex carbohydrates, found in whole grains, legumes, and vegetables, are digested more slowly, providing a more gradual increase in blood sugar and, importantly, a longer-lasting feeling of fullness which can help in overall calorie control.

The concept of the glycemic index (GI) is a tool developed to help decipher this dynamic. Foods with a high GI cause a rapid rise in blood glucose levels, while those with a low GI have a slower, more controlled effect. Learning to choose lower GI foods and combining them intelligently with proteins and fats can enrich your dietary palette without compromising blood sugar control.

Moreover, understanding the fiber factor further enhances our strategic approach to carbohydrates. Dietary fiber, a type of carbohydrate that the body can't digest, plays a crucial role in diabetes management. Soluble fiber, for example, can help to slow down the absorption of sugar, improving blood sugar levels. It also aids in lowering cholesterol and providing a sense of fullness, which can prevent overeating. Foods like oatmeal, apples, and carrots are rich in soluble fiber and can be fundamental components of your diet.

As we navigate these choices, it becomes clear that not all carbohydrates are created equal. Embracing whole, unprocessed options like vegetables, fruits, and whole grains can have a profound impact on managing diabetes. These foods not only maintain lower blood sugar levels but also enrich your body with vitamins, minerals, and antioxidants necessary for overall health.

Yet, the shift to a low-carb diet can seem daunting. It's common to feel restricted or overwhelmed by the need to scrutinize every food choice. But rather than viewing it as a limitation, let's see it as an exploration. Each meal is an opportunity to discover what combinations not only keep your blood sugar in check but also awaken your taste buds. Pairing a high-carb food with a healthy fat or a protein can balance your meal's impact on your blood sugar. For example, enjoying a slice of whole-grain bread with avocado or a small apple with a handful of almonds.

This approach extends to other areas of life. Social gatherings, holidays, and dining out, traditionally challenging situations for those managing diabetes, can now be navigated with greater confidence. By understanding the nature of carbohydrates and their effects, you can make informed choices that align with your health goals, allowing you to engage fully in every aspect of life without fear of losing control over your diabetes.

Incorporating these strategies does not only provide control over diabetes but also contributes to a richer, fuller life. The goal is not just to manage blood sugar levels but to enhance your overall wellness through mindful eating—an appreciation not only for the foods you eat but how they contribute to your life's quality.

Hence, consider carbohydrates not as mere numbers to be tallied or avoided but as part of a broader narrative of health and vitality. With this balanced, informed perspective, managing your diabetes can become not only easier but also more enjoyable. As you turn each page of your dietary journey, remember that knowledge is the flavor that makes all the difference—empowering you to craft a life not defined by diabetes but enriched by the choices you make daily.

The Importance of Protein in a Diabetic Diet

Protein, the building block of life, occupies a pivotal role in everyone's diet, particularly for those navigating life with diabetes after 50. This macronutrient, celebrated for its strength-building and appetite-regulating benefits, is versatile enough to support bodily functions and manage blood sugar levels robustly.

The significance of protein in a diabetic diet goes beyond its well-touted role in muscle repair and growth. One of its lesser-known yet critically important functions is its minimal impact on blood sugar levels compared to carbohydrates. When you consume protein, it does not directly translate into glucose in your bloodstream, a process beneficial for managing diabetes, as it avoids the sharp spikes in blood sugar that carbohydrates can induce.

However, the role of protein extends further, influencing how the body manages and utilizes insulin. Adequate protein intake can improve insulin sensitivity, which means your body can manage blood sugar more effectively. This is particularly vital for those managing Type 2 diabetes, where insulin resistance is a prevalent challenge. By improving insulin sensitivity, proteins help maintain a stable metabolic environment, reducing the risk of diabetes-related complications.

Another compelling attribute of protein in the diabetic diet is its effect on satiety—the feeling of being full. Protein-rich meals contribute to a longer-lasting satiety, which helps prevent overeating, a significant benefit when looking to manage or reduce weight, a common concern for those diagnosed with diabetes. Managing weight effectively can lead to improved glycemic control, thus reducing the severity of diabetes symptoms.

Diverse sources of protein also mean that individuals can tailor their diets in a way that respects their culinary preferences and ethical or health-related restrictions. Animal-based proteins such as chicken, fish, and dairy products provide high-quality proteins replete with essential amino acids. On the other hand, plant-based proteins found in beans, lentils, and tofu are invaluable options for those pursuing vegetarian or vegan lifestyles, proving that managing diabetes does not mean compromising on personal food ethics.

It's important to consider that not all protein sources are equal, particularly when it comes to managing diabetes. For example, red and processed meats, although high in protein, are also associated with cardiovascular risks and should be consumed with caution, particularly for those already managing cardiovascular symptoms alongside diabetes. Choosing lean protein sources, or integrating plant-based proteins, can offer the necessary nutrients without additional health risks.

The synergy between protein and other nutrients in meal planning also holds significant implications for blood sugar management. Combining protein with fiber-rich carbohydrates can slow the release of glucose into the blood, providing a steady energy release and maintaining stable blood sugar levels. Such combinations are not just beneficial—they are also delicious. The blending of flavors and textures can transform a meal from mere sustenance to a delightful culinary experience that also supports your health goals.

There's an art to incorporating the right amount of protein in one's diet, especially when considering the increased protein needs of older adults, including those over 50. Aging bodies process protein less efficiently, and muscle mass tends to decline, making it even more essential to ensure adequate protein intake.

Understanding these needs isn't just about meeting recommended dietary allowances—it's about creating a harmonious balance that supports your body's unique requirements. This balance is crucial not just for managing existing health conditions but also for preventing further complications, a common concern as bodies age and health conditions evolve.

Reflecting on your eating habits to incorporate adequate protein is akin to fine-tuning a musical instrument. Each meal becomes an opportunity to optimize how your body functions, helping to control not just diabetes, but also enhancing overall vitality and well-being.

The importance of protein in the diet underscores a broader principle integral to managing life with diabetes: dietary choices must support holistic health goals. Each nutrient, each meal choice, each day of eating right, acts like a thread in a larger tapestry, depicting a lifestyle oriented toward sustained health and wellness.

By understanding how to use protein efficiently and effectively within a dietary plan, individuals with diabetes can ensure they're not just surviving but thriving. The conversation around protein is more than just about consumption; it's about constructing a lifestyle that enriches, sustains, and nurtures, allowing every individual to lead a life that is as full and vibrant as the variety of proteins on their plate.

Healthy Fats: How They Help in Blood Sugar Regulation

In the narrative of nutritional health, fats have often been depicted as dietary antagonists. However, as we navigate the complexities of a diabetes-friendly diet, it's essential to reshape our understanding of fats—more specifically, healthy fats—and recognize their role not only as nutritional necessities but as allies in blood sugar regulation and overall wellness.

For ages, fats were mostly shunned, believed to be the primary culprits behind weight gain and heart diseases. Yet, modern science has painted a more nuanced picture, revealing that healthy fats are, in fact, crucial to our diet. They aid in the absorption of vitamins, provide us with energy, and importantly for those managing diabetes, help moderate blood sugar levels.

The key to understanding fats' impact on blood sugar lies in their relationship with digestion. Fats slow down the process by which the stomach empties, leading to a more gradual release of glucose into the bloodstream. This slower process reduces spikes in blood sugar, which is particularly beneficial for insulin management—a core concern for individuals with diabetes.

To incorporate healthy fats into your diet, it's vital to first identify them. Monounsaturated and polyunsaturated fats are considered heart-healthy options. Sources such as olive oil, avocados, nuts, and seeds not only contribute these beneficial fats but also enrich the diet with flavors that can make diabetic-friendly meals more enjoyable and satiating.

Moreover, recent studies suggest that omega-3 fatty acids, a type of polyunsaturated fat found abundantly in fatty fish like salmon and mackerel, have significant health benefits. Omega-3s are known to reduce inflammation, lower heart disease risk, and potentially aid in glucose regulation, making them an excellent addition to a diabetic diet.

However, while understanding which fats to embrace, it's equally crucial to know which to reduce. Saturated fats and trans fats, commonly found in butter, margarine, fast foods, and many processed options, should be limited. These fats can contribute to insulin resistance, an undesirable effect for anyone, but particularly those managing diabetes. Effectively, while not all fats are foes, some indeed are, and discerning their differences is critical.

This revelation about healthy fats invites us to rethink not just what we eat but how we prepare our foods. Cooking with oils rich in unsaturated fats, such as olive or canola oil, can transform a simple meal into both a healthful and delightful experience that supports your diabetes management goals. It's less about restricting your diet and more about reshaping it to include the right fats that promote both taste and health.

Incorporating healthy fats also means rethinking how we snack. Opting for nuts or seeds over chips or processed snacks can significantly enhance the quality of your diet, providing essential nutrients and fibers that promote satiety, reduce cravings, and help maintain stable glucose levels.

Yet, the role of fats extends beyond just nutritional input. Emotionally and psychologically, having a diet that includes flavorful and satisfying options like avocados, nuts, and olive oil can make the journey of managing diabetes more pleasant and sustainable. This positive psychological impact should not be underestimated, as emotional well-being is fundamentally connected to overall health, especially in managing chronic conditions like diabetes.

Integrating healthy fats shouldn't be a chore but a journey towards discovering meals and snacks that are as nutritious as they are satisfying. Think of each meal as a puzzle piece, where fats fit in to complete the picture of your daily nutritional needs, ensuring you're not just eating to survive but thriving on a diet that supports every aspect of your health.

Thus, the shift from viewing fats with suspicion to recognizing their value in a balanced diabetic diet marks a crucial step in managing diabetes effectively. This approach not only supports better blood sugar control but also enhances overall life quality, providing a fuller, more integrated method of health management where every calorie consumed serves a purpose towards greater wellness.

By redefining our relationship with fats and selecting the healthiest forms, we arm ourselves with the tools not just to manage diabetes, but to enjoy a richer, more flavorful life, underpinned by robust health and vitality. The narrative of fats in our diet is complex, yet abundantly clear—it's not about elimination, but about intelligent integration.

Essential Vitamins and Minerals for Diabetic Health

As we navigate the intricacies of managing diabetes, especially past the age of fifty, the focus often gravitates towards carbohydrates, fats, and proteins. However, the role of vitamins and minerals in diabetic health is equally pivotal, serving not just as mere footnotes in our dietary discussions but as fundamental components that can significantly influence blood sugar control and overall wellness.

Understanding the complex interplay of these micronutrients in managing diabetes involves delving into their specific functions and benefits. Each vitamin and mineral has a unique role, contributing to the body's ability to process glucose effectively, protect against oxidative stress, and maintain cellular health, which are all crucial for individuals managing diabetes.

Take magnesium, for instance. Found abundantly in leafy greens, nuts, and whole grains, magnesium aids in glucose metabolism and has been linked to improved insulin sensitivity. Low levels of magnesium have been associated with worse control of type 2 diabetes, highlighting the importance of this mineral in your daily intake.

Similarly, Vitamin D, often hailed as the 'sunshine vitamin,' is crucial for bone health and immune function but also plays a role in the pancreatic secretion of insulin. Research suggests that adequate levels of Vitamin D may enhance the body's ability to manage glucose levels effectively. This connection underscores the need for regular exposure to sunlight and potentially supplementing with Vitamin D, especially in individuals with diagnosed deficiencies or limited sun exposure.

Zinc, another essential trace mineral, is pivotal for the synthesis of insulin in the pancreas. It also plays a significant role in the storage and secretion of insulin, making it a critical component of a diabetes management plan. Regular consumption of zinc-rich foods like seafood, meat, seeds, and legumes can help maintain these essential processes.

Antioxidants such as vitamins C and E deserve mention too, as they combat oxidative stress — a condition diabetics are particularly prone to due to high blood glucose levels. This oxidative stress can damage cells and contribute to the complications associated with diabetes. Foods rich in these vitamins, like citrus fruits for Vitamin C and almonds for Vitamin E, can provide natural protection against such damage.

The role of vitamin B complex, including vitamins like B1 (thiamine), B6, and B12, in diabetes cannot be underestimated. These vitamins help convert food into energy and maintain proper nerve function. People with diabetes often have higher requirements for some of these nutrients, as they can be lost more frequently due to increased urination when blood sugar levels are high. Ensuring adequate intake of these vitamins through diet or supplements can help reduce symptoms of neuropathy, a common diabetic complication.

The challenge often lies not just in understanding the importance of these micronutrients, but in integrating them into a daily eating plan without feeling overwhelmed. It's about creating a balance, incorporating a variety of nutrients in the diet through a colorful palette of foods. Think of your plate as a canvas, each meal an opportunity to paint with vibrant veggies, fruits, lean proteins, whole grains, and healthy fats, all contributing to your micronutrient needs.

Moreover, while the focus is often on supplementation for getting these vital micronutrients, there is significant value in getting them from natural food sources. This approach not only ensures a broader intake of essential compounds but also benefits overall health due to the diverse range of nutrients present in whole foods.

Indeed, managing diabetes with a proper understanding of micronutrients can lead to more than just controlled blood sugar levels. It can enhance energy, boost mood, and improve overall physical and mental health. It embodies a holistic approach to diabetes management, where the goal is not just to live with the condition but to thrive.

By thoroughly integrating essential vitamins and minerals into everyday meals, individuals with diabetes can create a robust defense against the typical complications associated with the condition, turning dietary management into a pathway for enhanced life quality. Through this nutrient-rich approach, the journey with diabetes becomes one of empowerment and health, filled not just with good food but also with vitality and wellness.

Foods to Embrace and Foods to Avoid

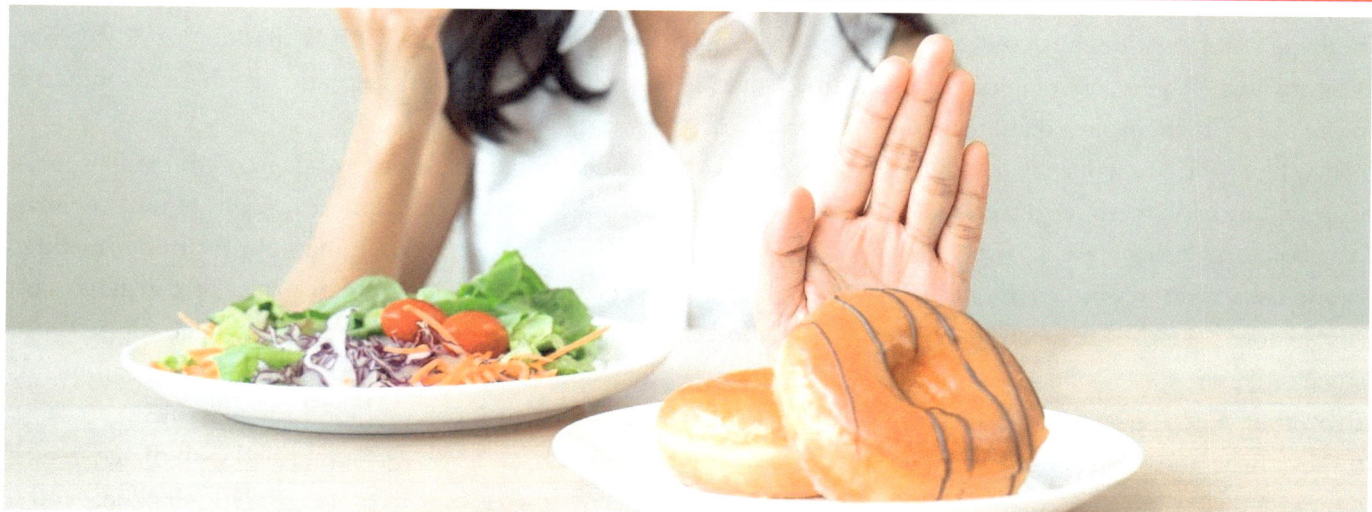

Embarking on a journey through the world of food when you're managing diabetes can feel like navigating a labyrinth. On one hand, certain foods serve as your allies, fortifying your health and keeping your blood sugars balanced. On the other, some foods pose challenges, threatening spikes and instability. Understanding this landscape is crucial, especially after reaching the golden age of fifty, when our bodies demand more attentive care.

Imagine walking through a vibrant market with stalls brimming with fresh produce: vivid greens, deep purples, and fiery reds. Each color not just a feast for the eyes but a signal of the nutritional treasures they hold. Foods rich in fiber like leafy greens, cruciferous vegetables, and legumes are your best friends. They are like the quiet neighbors who always support you—reliable, beneficial, and always there when you need them.

Contrast this with navigating a carnival, where every turn tempts you with sugary treats and ultra-processed foods—each one an adversary dressed in alluring colors and enchanting scents. While the immediate gratification might beckon, they are much like fair-weather friends, offering short-lived joy that could compromise long-term wellbeing.

This chapter invites you on a culinary exploration, guiding you through a landscape dotted with wholesome choices while cautioning you against the less favorable. It's about finding pleasure in the foods that nourish you deeply, sustainably. We'll uncover the secrets to using spices, herbs, and healthy fats not just as ingredients, but as tools to enhance flavor without adding unnecessary sugar or carbohydrates. Navigating this world with knowledge and confidence transforms your diet from a list of restrictions to a canvas of colorful, creative opportunities for nourishment. It's not merely about avoiding risks, but embracing a new, vibrant way of eating that enhances your health and your life. Join me in discovering how to make your diet a powerful ally in managing diabetes.

Low-Carb Foods for Blood Sugar Control

Navigating the world of a low-carb diet for effective blood sugar control can be akin to mastering the art of balance in a tightrope walk. Each food choice can significantly impact your blood glucose levels, making it essential to select those that help maintain stability. Let's explore the realm of low-carb foods, not just as dietary options, but as fundamental elements that support your health in managing diabetes after fifty.

Imagine each meal as an opportunity to positively influence your blood sugar levels. Integrating low-carb foods into your diet is not just about reduction; it's about making strategic choices that satisfy, nourish, and stabilize. It's important to approach these choices with curiosity and an open mind, diving into a diverse world of flavors and textures that perhaps you haven't explored before.

Vegetables: The backbone of any nutritious diet, particularly in managing diabetes, is a wide array of vegetables. Picture your plate, half-full of colorful, fibrous, and low-carb vegetables like spinach, kale, broccoli, and bell peppers. These foods are not just low in carbohydrates but are high in fiber, which helps slow down glucose absorption and prevent blood sugar spikes.

Proteins: Lean proteins such as chicken breast, turkey, fish, and plant-based proteins like tofu and tempeh play a pivotal role. They do not directly impact your blood sugar levels, making them a safe and essential component of your meal planning. When you incorporate a serving of protein in your meals, you're not only satiating hunger but also enabling your body to repair and build tissue without affecting your glucose levels.

Healthy Fats: While fats are often vilified, healthy fats are exceptionally beneficial, especially in a low-carb diet. Foods rich in omega-3 fatty acids like salmon, chia seeds, flaxseeds, and walnuts not only help sustain your feeling of fullness but also support cardiovascular health—a concern for many with diabetes.

Nuts and Seeds: These are remarkable not just for their crunch but also for their role in blood sugar control. Almonds, walnuts, and chia seeds offer a great combination of fats, protein, and fiber. They're like the Swiss Army knife in your dietary toolkit—versatile and effective.

Dairy and Dairy Alternatives: Choosing low-carb options in dairy or its alternatives can also support blood sugar management. Greek yogurt, for instance, provides a creamy texture and a good protein source, while being relatively low in carbs. It's important, however, to opt for plain versions without added sugars—it's the hidden sugars in flavored yogurts that can send your blood sugar soaring.

Fruits: While fruits are often seen as sugar-laden, choosing low glycemic index fruits can allow you to enjoy the sweetness without the guilt. Berries such as strawberries, blueberries, and blackberries, and fruits like apples and pears with their skins on, offer fiber and nutrients while keeping carbohydrate intake in check.

Embedding these food groups into your daily routine involves creativity and exploring new culinary avenues. Picture redesigning your morning breakfast where instead of a high-carb bagel or cereal, you opt for a spinach and mushroom omelet topped with avocado—a meal high in protein and healthy fats, keeping your morning blood sugar stable.

For lunch, envision a vibrant salad with mixed greens, cherry tomatoes, slices of grilled chicken, and a sprinkle of nuts, dressed in olive oil and vinegar. Such a meal not only satiates but also aligns with your low-carb goals without compromising on taste or nutrition.

The dinner could be a serving of grilled salmon or tofu, sautéed green beans, and a side of cauliflower rice—a perfect low-carb substitute for traditional rice, making your meal hearty and fulfilling without a carb overload.

Undoubtedly, transitioning to a low-carb lifestyle requires adjustments, but it's hardly about subtraction. It's about substituting wisely and finding pleasure in the abundance of options available that align with your health goals. You aren't just reducing carbs; you're reinventing your taste palette, exploring textures and flavors in a way that elevates your meals from mere nourishment to an enjoyable culinary journey that supports your health.

Managing diabetes, especially post-50, should not be a daunting task laden with restrictions. It's about embracing a lifestyle that includes a plethora of satisfying, nutritious, and stabilizing foods. It's about making every meal an opportunity to nurture your body, ensuring each dish brings you flavor and joy without compromising your health. Embarking on this low-carb journey can be one of the most empowering steps towards a balanced, healthful life, enabling you to tackle diabetes with confidence and gusto.

Fiber-Rich Foods: How They Benefit Diabetes

Unfolding the narrative of dietary fibers in the management of diabetes is almost like reading a thrilling novel where the hero, fiber, plays a critical role in maintaining health—especially after the age of fifty when dietary needs become all the more crucial. The incorporation of fiber-rich foods into your diet isn't just beneficial; it's transformative, offering multiple health advantages, particularly effective blood sugar control and cardiovascular health—a boon to any diabetic regimen.

The scene opens with understanding what exactly dietary fiber is. It's a type of carbohydrate that the body can't digest. While most carbs are broken down into sugar molecules, fiber passes through the body undigested, aiding digestive health and more, which brings us to its first role in managing diabetes.

Picture this: It's a typical morning, and you start your day with a bowl of oatmeal topped with fresh berries. Here, fiber enters the scene, acting not just as a protagonist to your breakfast plate, but also to your health. The soluble fiber in oatmeal forms a gel-like substance as it digests, slowing down the absorption of sugars in the bloodstream. This process helps maintain steady blood sugar levels, reducing the sudden spikes that are so common in diabetes management.

Now, let's journey through a day filled with fiber. For lunch, a quinoa salad with mixed vegetables like carrots, broccoli, and sweet peas, each crunchy forkful not only satisfying your taste buds but also working to control your appetite. High-fiber foods such as these are more filling, which helps curb overeating—particularly beneficial when maintaining a healthy weight is crucial for effective diabetes management.

The tale continues into the afternoon. Snacking becomes less about indulgence and more about strategic choices. Almonds and chia seeds are the snacks of choice, low in carbs but high in fiber, keeping you full, and keeping your blood sugar levels stable until dinner.

As the sun sets and dinner approaches, imagine a plate of grilled salmon with a side of Brussels sprouts and a lentil pilaf. The insoluble fiber in the lentils and Brussels sprouts doesn't dissolve, instead, it adds bulk to your stool, which aids in regular digestion and prevents the constipation often seen in diabetic patients due to certain medications.

The narrative of fiber doesn't just end with digestion and blood sugar control. It has a broader impact, particularly on heart health. Considering diabetes increases the risk of heart disease, fiber's role extends to managing cholesterol levels. The soluble fiber found in beans, oats, flaxseeds, and apples, helps reduce low-density lipoprotein (LDL), or "bad" cholesterol levels. It's like the hero's sidekick, supporting the fight against potential villains—heart disease and stroke.

Fiber's benefits reach even further, extending to the realm of gut health. A thriving community of gut flora is a cornerstone of good health. High-fiber foods act as prebiotics, feeding the good bacteria in your gut, which helps with inflammation, improves gastrointestinal health, and ultimately, aids in better overall health management.

But how does one ensure enough fiber intake? It's in the mindful integration of these foods throughout your daily meals, understanding which choices pack the most punch, and creatively incorporating them into your diet. The attention should not solely be on the obvious choices like fruits and vegetables. Consider too the less thought of, like pulses – beans, lentils, chickpeas. These are not only high in fiber but are also excellent protein sources, giving a double win for those managing diabetes.

In envisioning a day or even a life packed with fiber, we aren't just looking at managing diabetes effectively. We're looking at enhancing life's quality, maintaining independence, and relishing food that's as satisfying as it is nourishing. The story of fiber is one of empowerment, enabling you to take control of your health narrative with informed, flavorful choices that help maintain not just your blood sugar but also your zest for life.

So as you turn each page of your day, remember that adding fiber-rich foods is like adding chapters to your life's story, each page enriched with health, flavor, and the joys of eating well. It's not merely about living longer; it's about living healthier, fuller, and more vibrant every day.

Foods to Avoid: High-Sugar and Processed Items

In any narrative, there are characters that, while charismatic, can lead our hero astray. In the tale of managing diabetes post-50, high-sugar and heavily processed foods play the part of the enchanting but dangerous sirens, luring you with instant gratification while compromising long-term health goals.

These food villains, often cloaked in convenient packaging and promising irresistible flavors, are staples in many diets but carry implications particularly impactful for those managing diabetes. Understanding the nature of these foods and their effects can guide you to make safer, healthier choices that support your dietary aims.

High-sugar items are among the chief culprits in disrupting blood sugar levels. Sugar, particularly refined sugar found in sodas, desserts, and snacks, can cause blood glucose levels to spike rapidly. This surge forces the body to process a large amount of sugar quickly, a process that, over time, can lead to insulin resistance—a condition that is central to the development of type 2 diabetes.

Visualize walking down a supermarket aisle, bombarded by colorful packages of cookies, cakes, and candies. Their appeal is undeniable, but beneath their vibrant exteriors lies a less appealing truth: these are foods with high glycemic indices which contribute to rapid rises and falls in blood sugar levels, leading to energy crashes that can affect your mood, your daily performance, and significantly, your metabolic health.

Processed foods extend beyond just sweets. Many packaged snacks, instant meals, and fast foods undergo extensive processing, stripping away beneficial nutrients while adding preservatives, unhealthy fats, and hidden sugars. The risk? These foods, while convenient, increase caloric intake without offering nutritional value, compounding challenges in managing a healthy weight—a key aspect of diabetes management.

One might ask, how can these food villains be so pervasive? The answer often lies in their design. Processed foods are typically engineered for long shelf life and palatability, not for health. They often contain high amounts of sodium, trans fats, and sugars to enhance taste and texture, which over time can lead not just to diabetes complications but also to heart disease and other health issues.

To illustrate, imagine your dietary journey as a scenic path in a beautiful, expansive garden. Each step on this path contributes to your health journey. Now, imagine that path lined with traps hidden amidst the greenery—these are processed foods. Each step you take on these traps can potentially cause you to stumble or fall, deviating from your path of managing diabetes effectively.

Furthermore, the impact of these foods is not limited to physical aspects alone. Diabetes management also encompasses mental and emotional health. Consuming high amounts of sugar and unhealthy fats has been linked to mood swings, depression, and decreased cognitive function. Thus, the consumption of these foods can become a cyclical enemy: they may temporarily boost mood with a sugar rush, but this is often followed by a crash, leading to further cravings and a deeper plunge into undesirable dietary habits.

In steering clear of these risky dietary choices, consider the role of awareness and education. Recognizing the content and makeup of your food by reading labels is a form of empowerment. Knowledge allows for informed decisions, helping you avoid hidden sugars and excessive sodium, which are often masked under less known names.

The approach, therefore, involves more than mere avoidance; it's about making conscious choices. Opt for whole, unprocessed foods when possible—fruits, vegetables, lean proteins, and whole grains. These are foods that truly nourish and sustain, providing lasting energy and stabilizing blood sugar levels.

In conclusion, managing diabetes effectively after 50 isn't just about avoiding what harms you but also embracing what heals you. It's about making choices that enhance your well-being so that your diet doesn't just keep you away from harm, but actively promotes better, healthier living. Your diet, much like any good story, should be filled with characters that support the protagonist—you—in your journey towards health and vitality.

Navigating Processed Foods: Understanding Labels and Hidden Sugars

Embarking on a mixed journey in the world of processed foods, the importance of understanding food labels emerges as a crucial navigational tool. This journey is less about avoiding all processed foods—many of which can include basic, beneficial processing—and more about learning to identify those products that carry hidden, potentially harmful ingredients like added sugars and unhealthy fats.

Venturing into the grocery store can be likened to setting out on an expedition. Each aisle and every shelf is stocked with promises of nourishment, convenience, and taste. Yet beneath the appealing packaging and alluring descriptions, there lies an array of complex labels that often conceal more than they reveal. Becoming adept at decoding these labels is akin to mastering a new language—a language essential for maintaining health, particularly in managing diabetes.

Start with the basics: understanding the list of ingredients. Ingredients on a food label are listed in order of quantity—from the highest to the lowest. This simple yet profound piece of information can be an eye-opener, especially when sugars or unhealthy fats appear near the top of this list, signaling their high concentration.

But sugars have their disguises, many names that sound less alarming. Terms like sucrose, glucose, high-fructose corn syrup, maltose, dextrose, cane juice, and syrup are just a few. Recognizing these terms is pivotal. Each term signals added sugars that, while they may add appeal to taste buds, disrupt the careful blood sugar balance essential for managing diabetes.

Imagine walking down a cereal aisle, picking up a box that claims to be a "healthy, whole-grain" breakfast option. A quick glance at the nutrition facts might show an acceptable amount of sugar. However, a more thorough reading of the ingredients may reveal sugars hidden under less recognized aliases. This deeper looking reveals the true nature of the product beyond the surface-level claims.

Another critical aspect is the nutritional content label, particularly the section that lists total carbohydrates, which includes all sugars, fibers, and starches. For someone managing diabetes, understanding the balance between these elements is key. Fiber, for instance, mitigates the impact of net carbs on blood sugar levels and can balance out the negative effects of other carbohydrates.

The label also reveals the presence of trans fats—often found in processed snacks, baked goods, and fried foods—which should be avoided as they are harmful to heart health, an important consideration for anyone, but particularly for those over fifty and managing diabetes.

Consider a scenario where you're assessing a packaged meal for dinner. The front of the package boasts "low-fat" and "reduced-sodium," criteria that might initially seem to align with dietary guidelines. Yet, on closer inspection, the list of ingredients might show hidden sugars and a chemical composition of preservatives that negate any potential benefit that could have come from low fat or sodium.

Understanding these labels also means paying attention to serving sizes, which can often be misleading. What might appear as a reasonable amount of sugar or sodium per serving can quickly become excessive if the actual serving size is smaller than the amount you would typically consume.

Navigating this complex landscape requires a sharp eye and an informed mind. Education about these subtleties helps turn each grocery shopping trip into an empowered decision-making process. You learn not just to see what is immediately evident but to understand what lies beneath, choosing foods that support your health goals rather than hinder them.

Thus armed with knowledge and discernment, you can walk through any grocery store with confidence, picking items off the shelf not just based on external appearances or vague health claims, but based on a thorough understanding of their contents. This skill enhances not only your ability to manage diabetes effectively but also your overall quality of life, granting you the freedom to enjoy a variety of foods while keeping your health on track.

In this way, the grocery store transforms from a minefield of potential dietary pitfalls into a treasure trove of nourishment. Each label read correctly is a step forward in your health journey, a small victory in managing your diabetes with knowledge and confidence. By mastering the language of labels, you turn processed foods from potential enemies into allies in your quest for health.

FOODS TO EMBRACE FOR DIABETICS OVER 50:

1. **Leafy greens (spinach, kale)** – Low in carbs, high in nutrients.
2. **Broccoli** – Rich in fiber, helps control blood sugar.
3. **Cauliflower** – Low-carb alternative, high in fiber.
4. **Brussels sprouts** – Low in carbs, high in vitamins.
5. **Zucchini** – Low in carbs and versatile.
6. **Cucumbers** – Low-carb, hydrating vegetable.
7. **Green beans** – Low in carbs and fiber-rich.
8. **Asparagus** – Low in carbs, high in vitamins.
9. **Bell peppers** – Low in sugar, high in vitamin C.
10. **Tomatoes** – Low in carbs, high in antioxidants.
11. **Avocados** – High in healthy fats, good for blood sugar control.
12. **Berries (strawberries, blueberries, raspberries)** – Low in sugar, high in fiber and antioxidants.
13. **Chia seeds** – High in fiber and omega-3s.
14. **Flaxseeds** – Rich in fiber and healthy fats.
15. **Walnuts** – Good source of omega-3s.
16. **Almonds** – High in protein and fiber.
17. **Pumpkin seeds** – Rich in magnesium, helps regulate blood sugar.
18. **Sunflower seeds** – Good source of healthy fats.
19. **Olive oil** – Healthy fat, good for heart health.
20. **Coconut oil (in moderation)** – Contains medium-chain triglycerides (MCTs).
21. **Fatty fish (salmon, mackerel, sardines)** – Rich in omega-3 fatty acids, good for inflammation.
22. **Chicken breast (skinless)** – High in protein, low in carbs.
23. **Turkey breast** – Lean protein, low in carbs.
24. **Eggs** – High-quality protein, helps keep you full.
25. **Greek yogurt (unsweetened)** – High in protein, low in sugar.
26. **Cottage cheese (low-fat)** – High in protein, low-carb option.
27. **Tofu** – High in protein, plant-based option.
28. **Tempeh** – Fermented, high in protein and fiber.
29. **Lentils** – High in fiber, helps stabilize blood sugar.
30. **Chickpeas** – Fiber-rich, low glycemic index.
31. **Black beans** – High in fiber and protein.
32. **Quinoa** – High-protein, whole grain alternative.
33. **Steel-cut oats** – High in fiber, slow to digest.
34. **Barley** – High in fiber, can help with blood sugar control.
35. **Brown rice (in moderation)** – Whole grain, better alternative to white rice.
36. **Sweet potatoes** – High in fiber, lower glycemic index than white potatoes.
37. **Butternut squash** – Nutrient-dense, good for blood sugar.
38. **Mushrooms** – Low in carbs, high in nutrients.

39. **Garlic** – May help improve blood sugar levels.

40. **Onions** – Low in carbs, adds flavor without sugar.

41. **Extra-virgin olive oil** – Healthy fat, promotes heart health.

42. **Herbs (basil, parsley, cilantro)** – Adds flavor without calories or carbs.

43. **Spices (turmeric, cinnamon)** – Anti-inflammatory, can help regulate blood sugar.

44. **Green tea** – May help improve insulin sensitivity.

45. **Herbal teas (peppermint, chamomile)** – No sugar, calming.

46. **Water** – Essential for health, calorie-free.

47. **Dark chocolate (85% cocoa or higher, in moderation)** – Low sugar, rich in antioxidants.

48. **Coconut flour** – Low-carb, gluten-free alternative for baking.

49. **Almond flour** – Low-carb, gluten-free flour alternative.

50. **Apple cider vinegar** – May help lower blood sugar after meals.

Foods to Avoid for Diabetics Over 50:

1. **White bread** – High in refined carbs, spikes blood sugar.
2. **Pastries (donuts, croissants, etc.)** – Loaded with sugar and unhealthy fats.
3. **Sugary cereals** – High in sugar, low in fiber.
4. **Regular soda** – Contains high amounts of sugar.
5. **Fruit-flavored yogurt (with added sugars)** – High in sugar, low in protein.
6. **White rice** – High in refined carbs, can cause blood sugar spikes.
7. **Candy bars** – High sugar and unhealthy fats.
8. **Sugary desserts (cakes, cookies)** – High sugar and refined carbs.
9. **Ice cream** – High in sugar and unhealthy fats.
10. **Fruit juices (with added sugar)** – High in sugar, causes blood sugar spikes.
11. **Processed meats (bacon, sausage)** – High in sodium and unhealthy fats.
12. **French fries** – Deep-fried and high in carbs.
13. **Chips (potato chips, tortilla chips)** – High in sodium and unhealthy fats.
14. **Canned fruits in syrup** – High in added sugar.
15. **Pancakes with syrup** – High in refined carbs and sugar.
16. **Flavored coffee drinks** – High in sugar.
17. **Energy drinks** – High in sugar and caffeine.
18. **Sweetened iced tea** – High in sugar.
19. **Packaged snack cakes** – High sugar and processed ingredients.
20. **Milkshakes** – High sugar and unhealthy fats.
21. **BBQ sauce (with high sugar content)** – Loaded with sugar.
22. **Ketchup (high sugar)** – Contains added sugars.
23. **Maple syrup** – Pure sugar, spikes blood sugar levels.
24. **Honey** – Natural but still high in sugar.
25. **Agave syrup** – High in fructose, can raise blood sugar.
26. **White pasta** – High in refined carbs.
27. **Deep-fried foods** – High in unhealthy fats.
28. **Bagels** – High in refined carbs, causes blood sugar spikes.
29. **Pizza (with thick crust)** – High in refined carbs and unhealthy fats.
30. **Sweetened granola** – High in sugar.
31. **Frozen dinners (high in sodium and sugars)** – Often contain hidden sugars.
32. **Margarine (with trans fats)** – Harmful fats that can worsen health conditions.
33. **Full-fat dairy (like cream)** – High in unhealthy fats.
34. **Sugar-coated nuts** – High in sugar.
35. **Dried fruits (with added sugar)** – Natural sugars are concentrated.
36. **Alcoholic cocktails** – High sugar content.
37. **Jams and jellies** – High sugar, even in small servings.
38. **Canned soups (high in sodium)** – Hidden sugars and sodium.
39. **Sweetened peanut butter** – Added sugars.
40. **Processed cheese** – High in unhealthy fats.
41. **High-sugar protein bars** – Often loaded with sugar.

42. **Commercial salad dressings (with added sugars)** – Hidden sugar.

43. **Canned beans (with added sugar or salt)** – Check for added sugars.

44. **Glazed ham** – High in sugar from the glaze.

45. **Biscuits** – High in refined carbs and fats.

46. **Syrup-covered waffles** – High sugar and refined carbs.

47. **Commercial smoothies** – Often loaded with added sugars.

48. **Instant noodles** – High in sodium and carbs.

49. **Regular crackers** – High in refined carbs.

50. **Sugary muffins** – High in sugar and refined carbs.

BREAKFAST

Good morning! Imagine starting your day with not just any meal, but one that fuels your body, stabilizes your blood sugar, and sets a positive tone for the rest of your waking hours. In this chapter, we delve into breakfasts that tick all these boxes—satisfying, simple to prepare, and splendidly suited to managing diabetes after 50.

Breakfast, often dubbed the most important meal of the day, holds particular significance for those managing diabetes. A robust morning meal can mitigate the blood glucose spikes that might occur later in the day and help maintain your energy levels. However, the typical breakfast fare—think pancakes dripping with syrup, or heaping servings of sugary cereals—poses a challenge for anyone conscious about carbohydrate intake. Here, we redefine breakfast with options designed to satisfy both your palate and your health requirements.

In our journey, we tackle two main challenges: maintaining a low-carb regimen and keeping morning prep effortless and enjoyable. Our recipes are structured to avoid monotonous dietary routines—imagine savoring almond flour pancakes topped with a berry compote or digging into a savory spinach and feta omelet. And yes, these are meals that can be whipped up with minimal fuss, keeping in mind that your morning is as precious as your health.

Each recipe in this section not only meets your dietary needs but also caters to your taste for variety and flavor. They are crafted to ensure that you never feel deprived but rather empowered, enjoying every breakfast as if it were a treat—indulgent yet incredibly in line with your health goals.

So, set aside your worries about post-breakfast blood sugar spikes. With the right ingredients and a few key techniques that we'll explore together, you'll see how comforting and beneficial a well-planned diabetic-friendly breakfast can be. Let's embrace these mornings with enthusiasm and a promise for a healthier day ahead!

BROCCOLI AND FETA OMELET

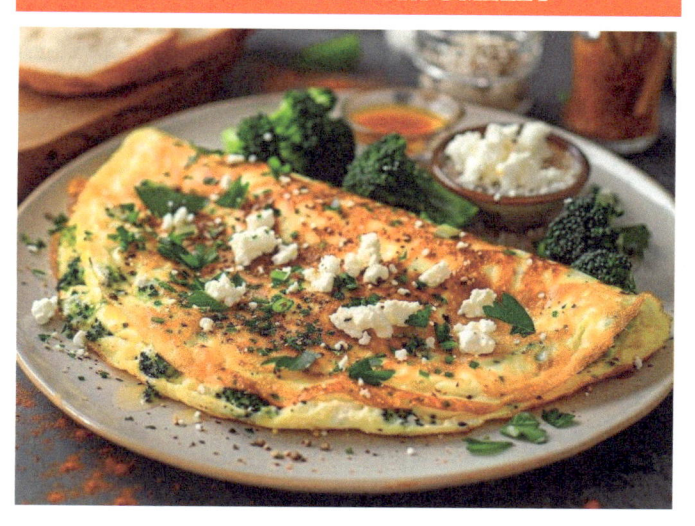

Preparation Time: 5 min
Cooking Time: 10 min
Servings: 1 Serv.
Glycemic Index: Low(~45)
Ingredients:

- 3 eggs, whisked
- 1 C. broccoli, finely chopped
- ¼ C. feta cheese, crumbled
- 1 Tbsp olive oil
- Salt and pepper to taste

Directions:

1. Preheat your nonstick skillet over medium heat and add olive oil
2. Add chopped broccoli and sauté until slightly tender
3. Pour in whisked eggs, sprinkle with salt and pepper
4. Let eggs set at the edges, then sprinkle feta over the top
5. Fold the omelet in half and cook until eggs are fully set
6. Serve hot

Tips:

- Opt for low-fat feta to reduce the overall fat content
- Accompany with a slice of whole-grain bread for added fiber

- A dash of hot sauce can enhance flavor without adding sugar

Nutritional Values: Calories: 320, Fat: 25g, Carbs: 6g, Protein: 20g, Sugar: 3g, Sodium: 640mg, Potassium: 300mg, Cholesterol: 370mg

CHIA AND ALMOND YOGURT PARFAIT

Preparation Time: 10 min
Cooking Time: none
Servings: 1
Glycemic Index: Low(~35)
Ingredients:

- 6 oz. Greek yogurt, unsweetened
- 2 Tbsp chia seeds
- 1/4 C. almonds, slivered
- 1/2 C. raspberries
- 1 tsp honey, optional
- 1/2 tsp vanilla extract

Directions:

1. In a bowl, mix Greek yogurt with vanilla extract and honey if using
2. Spoon half of the yogurt mixture into a glass
3. Add a layer of chia seeds followed by almonds and raspberries
4. Repeat the layers until all ingredients are used up
5. Chill in the refrigerator for a few minutes before serving to allow chia seeds to swell

Tips:

- Substitute raspberries with other low-GI berries like blackberries or strawberries for variety
- Enhance sweetness naturally by adding a dusting of cinnamon instead of honey
- To make it crunchier, toast the almonds slightly before adding to the parfait

Nutritional Values: Calories: 280, Fat: 15g, Carbs: 18g, Protein: 13g, Sugar: 8g, Sodium: 50mg, Potassium: 200mg, Cholesterol: 10mg

SPINACH AND MUSHROOM EGG MUFFINS

Preparation Time: 15 min
Cooking Time: 20 min
Servings: 6
Glycemic Index: Low(~50)
Ingredients:

- 6 eggs
- 1 C. spinach, chopped
- 1/2 C. mushrooms, diced
- 1/4 C. onions, finely chopped
- 1/4 C. cheddar cheese, shredded
- 1 Tbsp olive oil
- Salt and pepper to taste

Directions:

1. Preheat oven to 375°F (190°C)
2. In a skillet, heat olive oil and sauté onions, mushrooms, and spinach until tender
3. In a bowl, whisk eggs with salt and pepper, then stir in sautéed vegetables and cheddar cheese
4. Pour mixture into greased muffin tins, filling each cup about three-quarters full
5. Bake for 20 minutes or until muffins are set and lightly golden on top
6. Allow to cool slightly before serving

Tips:

- These muffins can be stored in the refrigerator for up to 4 days or frozen for longer storage
- Serve with a side of avocado for healthy fats
- Add a pinch of nutmeg or paprika for extra flavor

Nutritional Values: Calories: 120, Fat: 9g, Carbs: 3g, Protein: 8g, Sugar: 1g, Sodium: 125mg, Potassium: 150mg, Cholesterol: 195mg

CHIA AND HEMP SEED YOGURT PARFAIT

Preparation Time: 5 min
Cooking Time: none
Servings: 1
Glycemic Index: Low(~35)
Ingredients:

- 1 C. Greek yogurt, unsweetened
- 2 Tbsp chia seeds
- 1 Tbsp hemp seeds
- ½ C. blueberries
- ¼ C. almonds, slivered
- 1 tsp honey, optional
- 1 tsp cinnamon

Directions:
1. In a bowl, layer Greek yogurt with chia seeds, hemp seeds, and blueberries
2. Sprinkle slivered almonds and cinnamon on top
3. Drizzle with honey if desired
4. Serve immediately or chill in refrigerator for a thicker consistency

Tips:
- Opt for mixed berries for varied antioxidants
- Replace almonds with walnuts for a different texture and added omega-3s
- If avoiding honey, sweeten naturally with a bit of mashed banana

Nutritional Values: Calories: 310, Fat: 18g, Carbs: 23g, Protein: 20g, Sugar: 12g, Sodium: 85mg, Potassium: 250mg, Cholesterol: 10mg

TURMERIC TOFU SCRAMBLE

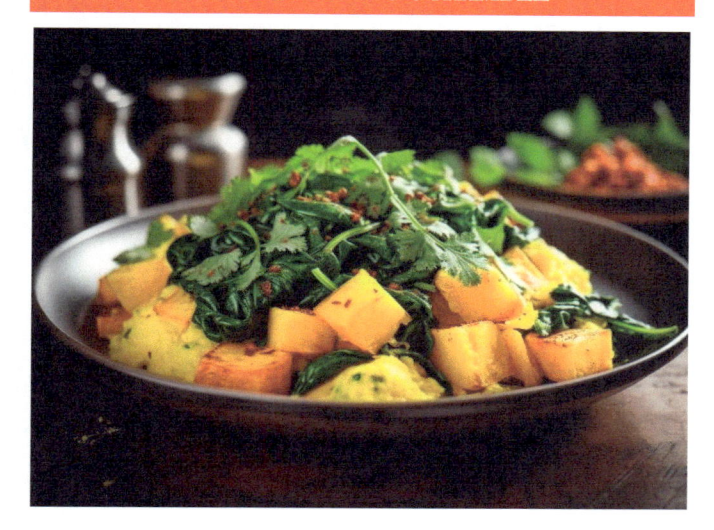

Preparation Time: 10 min
Cooking Time: 10 min
Servings: 2
Glycemic Index: Low(~50)
Ingredients:
- 14 oz. firm tofu, drained and crumbled
- 1 Tbsp olive oil
- ½ tsp turmeric
- ¼ tsp black pepper
- ½ C. red onion, finely chopped
- 1 C. kale, chopped
- 1 tsp garlic powder
- ½ tsp salt

Directions:
1. Heat olive oil in a skillet over medium heat
2. Add red onion and sauté until translucent
3. Stir in crumbled tofu, turmeric, black pepper, garlic powder, and salt
4. Cook for 7 min., stirring frequently
5. Mix in kale and cook until wilted, about 3 min. more
6. Serve warm

Tips:
- Add a splash of low-sodium soy sauce for extra flavor
- Serve with a slice of whole grain toast for added fiber
- Garnish with fresh parsley for a refreshing note

Nutritional Values: Calories: 220, Fat: 14g, Carbs: 10g, Protein: 19g, Sugar: 2g, Sodium: 330mg, Potassium: 300mg, Cholesterol: 0mg

SMOKED SALMON AND AVOCADO TARTINE

Preparation Time: 15 min
Cooking Time: none
Servings: 1
Glycemic Index: Low(~30)
Ingredients:
- 2 slices of low-carb whole grain bread, toasted
- 4 oz. smoked salmon
- 1 ripe avocado, sliced
- 1 Tbsp capers
- 1 Tbsp red onion, thinly sliced
- ½ lemon, juiced
- 1 tsp dill, fresh and chopped
- Black pepper to taste

Directions:
1. Arrange toasted bread on a plate
2. Layer smoked salmon and avocado slices on each piece
3. Top with capers, red onion, and a sprinkle of fresh dill
4. Finish with a drizzle of lemon juice and a pinch of black pepper
5. Serve immediately

Tips:
- Use a drizzle of extra virgin olive oil for added healthy fats
- Squeeze a bit of lemon on the avocado to prevent browning if serving later
- Pair with a side of cottage cheese for extra protein

Nutritional Values: Calories: 370, Fat: 22g, Carbs: 24g, Protein: 21g, Sugar: 4g, Sodium: 670mg, Potassium: 510mg, Cholesterol: 30mg

BERRY GINGER ZINGER SMOOTHIE

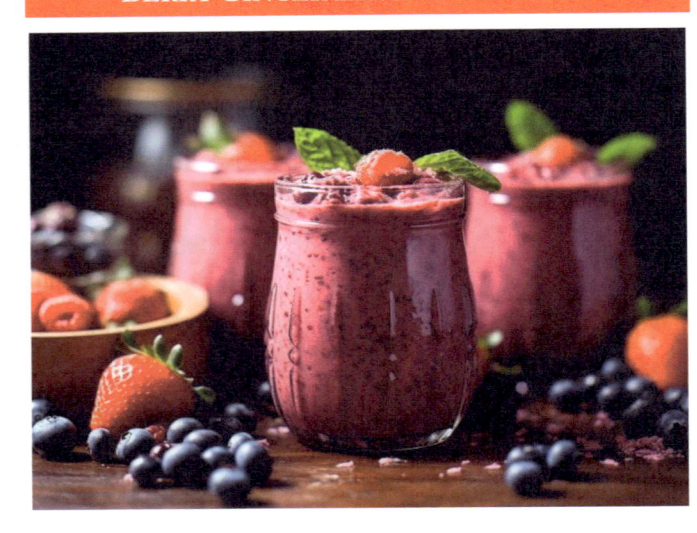

Preparation Time: 5 min
Cooking Time: none
Servings: 2
Glycemic Index: Low(~39)
Ingredients:
- 1 C. strawberries, fresh
- ½ C. blueberries, fresh
- 1 Tbsp ginger, freshly grated
- 1 C. Greek yogurt, unsweetened
- 1 Tbsp almond butter
- 1 C. ice
- 1 tsp lemon zest

Directions:
1. Combine strawberries, blueberries, ginger, Greek yogurt, almond butter, ice, and lemon zest in a blender
2. Blend until smooth
3. Pour into glasses and serve chilled

Tips:
- Add a scoop of protein powder for an extra boost
- Increase ginger if you prefer a spicier smoothie
- Substitute almond butter with cashew butter for a different flavor

Nutritional Values: Calories: 190, Fat: 8g, Carbs: 19g, Protein: 12g, Sugar: 10g, Sodium: 60mg, Potassium: 350mg, Cholesterol: 10mg

CUCUMBER MELON MEDLEY SHAKE

Preparation Time: 10 min
Cooking Time: none
Servings: 1
Glycemic Index: Low(~30)
Ingredients:
- ½ C. cucumber, peeled and chopped
- 1 C. cantaloupe, cubed
- ½ C. unsweetened almond milk
- ½ C. Greek yogurt, unsweetened
- 1 Tbsp flaxseeds, ground
- 1 tsp mint leaves, fresh
- ¼ C. ice cubes

Directions:
1. Place cucumber, cantaloupe, almond milk, Greek yogurt, flaxseeds, mint leaves, and ice cubes into a blender
2. Blend until smooth and frothy
3. Serve chilled in a tall glass

Tips:
- Incorporate a tablespoon of honey if a slight sweetness is desired
- Try adding a few drops of natural vanilla extract for fragrance
- Switch mint with basil for a different herbal note

Nutritional Values: Calories: 140, Fat: 3g, Carbs: 18g, Protein: 9g, Sugar: 13g, Sodium: 50mg, Potassium: 470mg, Cholesterol: 5mg

PEACHES AND CREAM OAT SHAKE

Preparation Time: 8 min
Cooking Time: none
Servings: 2
Glycemic Index: Low(~45)
Ingredients:
- 2 C. peaches, sliced and frozen

- 1 C. oat milk, unsweetened
- ½ C. cottage cheese, low-fat
- 1 Tbsp honey
- 1 tsp vanilla extract
- 1 Tbsp chia seeds
- ¼ C. ice cubes

Directions:
1. Add frozen peaches, oat milk, cottage cheese, honey, vanilla extract, chia seeds, and ice cubes to a blender
2. Blend until creamy
3. Serve immediately in chilled glasses

Tips:
- Experiment with different types of milk for variation
- Sprinkle ground cinnamon for a warm, comforting flavor
- A touch of nutmeg can elevate the creaminess

Nutritional Values: Calories: 210, Fat: 4g, Carbs: 32g, Protein: 10g, Sugar: 22g, Sodium: 65mg, Potassium: 550mg, Cholesterol: 5mg

CHIA AND COCONUT YOGURT PARFAIT

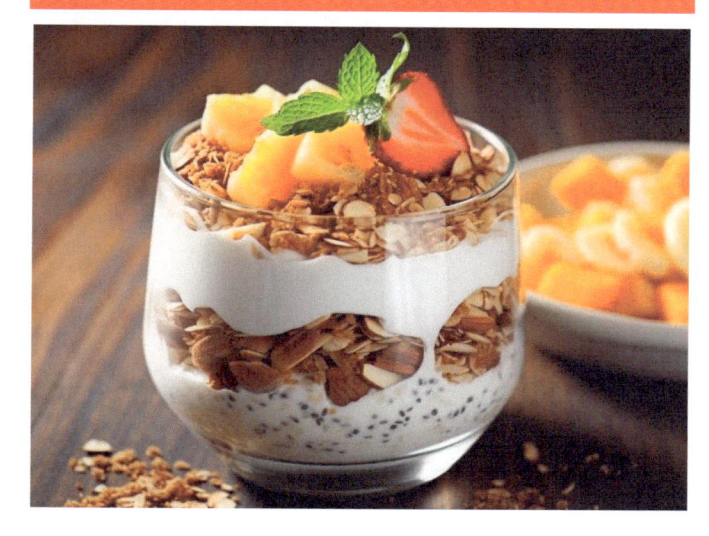

Preparation Time: 10 min
Cooking Time: none
Servings: 2
Glycemic Index: Low(~35)
Ingredients:
- ⅓ C. chia seeds
- 1 C. coconut yogurt, unsweetened
- ½ C. raspberries, fresh
- ¼ C. almonds, slivered
- 2 tsp honey, optional
- ¼ tsp vanilla extract
- 1 pinch cinnamon

Directions:
1. Mix chia seeds with coconut yogurt, honey, vanilla extract, and cinnamon in a bowl until well combined
2. Let the mixture sit for 5 minutes to allow chia seeds to swell
3. Layer the chia mixture with raspberries and slivered almonds in two serving glasses
4. Serve chilled or immediately

Tips:
- Prepare the night before and refrigerate for a grab-and-go breakfast
- Swap raspberries for mixed berries or seasonal fruits for variety
- To enhance sweetness, opt for a drizzle of agave nectar instead of honey

Nutritional Values: Calories: 295, Fat: 19g, Carbs: 23g, Protein: 8g, Sugar: 10g, Sodium: 35mg, Potassium: 270mg, Cholesterol: 0mg

SAVORY MUFFIN TIN OMELETTES

Preparation Time: 15 min
Cooking Time: 20 min
Servings: 6
Glycemic Index: Low(~50)
Ingredients:
- 6 eggs, well beaten
- ¼ C. bell peppers, diced
- ¼ C. onions, finely chopped
- ⅓ C. spinach, chopped
- ½ C. feta cheese, crumbled
- Salt to taste
- Black pepper to taste

Directions:
1. Preheat oven to 375°F (190°C)
2. Mix eggs, bell peppers, onions, spinach, feta cheese, salt, and pepper in a bowl
3. Grease a 6-cup muffin tin and evenly pour the egg mixture into each cup

4. Bake in preheated oven for 20 min or until the omelettes are set and lightly golden on top
5. Let cool for a few minutes before serving

Tips:
- Bake a batch ahead and store in the refrigerator for up to 4 days for easy reheat-and-go breakfasts
- Customize with different vegetables like mushrooms or zucchini for added flavor and nutrition
- Add a pinch of turmeric for anti-inflammatory benefits

Nutritional Values: Calories: 180, Fat: 12g, Carbs: 4g, Protein: 12g, Sugar: 2g, Sodium: 320mg, Potassium: 125mg, Cholesterol: 370mg

SMOKED SALMON AND HERB CREAM CHEESE WRAPS

Preparation Time: 10 min
Cooking Time: none
Servings: 4
Glycemic Index: Low(~45)
Ingredients:
- 4 whole grain tortillas
- 8 oz. smoked salmon
- ¼ C. cream cheese, light
- 1 Tbsp chives, finely chopped
- 1 Tbsp dill, freshly chopped
- 1 C. arugula
- Lemon zest from 1 lemon
- Salt and pepper to taste

Directions:
1. Spread each tortilla with cream cheese and sprinkle with chives, dill, and lemon zest
2. Top with smoked salmon slices and a handful of arugula
3. Season with salt and pepper
4. Roll up the tortillas tightly and slice into pinwheels or serve whole

Tips:
- Prepare wraps the night before and wrap tightly in foil to keep fresh for morning
- Substitute arugula with spinach for a milder flavor
- Enhance the wrap with thin slices of cucumber or radish for extra crunch

Nutritional Values: Calories: 300, Fat: 15g, Carbs: 20g, Protein: 20g, Sugar: 3g, Sodium: 670mg, Potassium: 360mg, Cholesterol: 50mg

LUNCH

Lunchtime presents a wonderful opportunity in the day of anyone managing diabetes, especially those of us who have celebrated more than a few birthdays. It's not just a break in the day; it's a chance to nourish our bodies, balance our blood sugar, and enjoy the flavors life has to offer—despite the dietary adjustments we might need to make.

Picture this: it's midday, and the usual hustle-bustle slows to a pause. This is the moment to step back and think about what your body truly needs. Gone are the hastily grabbed fast-food options that spike your sugar levels and leave you weary. Instead, imagine sitting down to a plate filled with vibrant, nourishing foods that not only taste wonderful but also support your health goals. A fresh, zesty salad topped with grilled chicken or perhaps a savory, low-carb wrap filled with an assortment of crisp, colorful vegetables and a smear of spicy mustard. Maybe it's a steaming bowl of vegetable-rich soup that warms your soul as much as it fills your stomach.

The recipes in this chapter are designed to be simple yet satisfying. They acknowledge your busy life and respect the culinary constraints of a low-carb, low-sugar diet without sacrificing flavor or fulfillment. Each meal is crafted to be prepared with ease, often with ingredients that are likely already in your pantry or can be easily found at your local grocery store.

Moreover, these meals are not just "good for a diabetic diet"—they are just plain good. They can be shared with friends and family without the slightest hesitation or need for explanation. After all, good health, like a good meal, is best when shared.

So, let's embrace lunch as more than just a meal. Let it be a celebration of health, of life, and of the joy to be found in eating well with diabetes.

SEARED TUNA AND AVOCADO SALAD

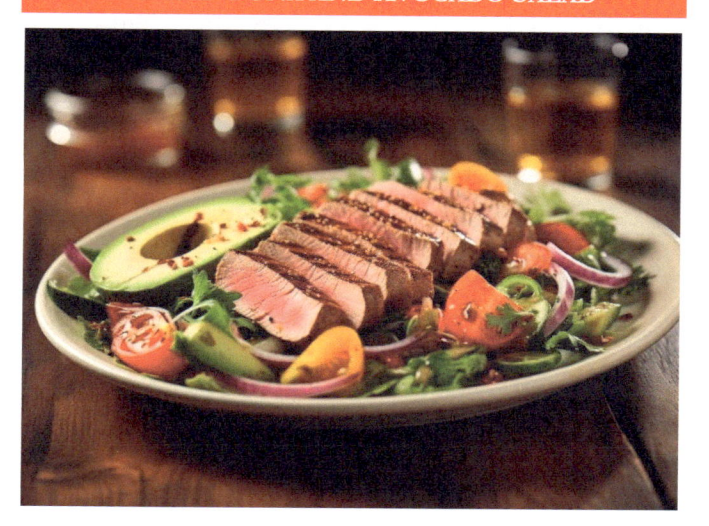

Preparation Time: 10 min
Cooking Time: 5 min
Servings: 2
Glycemic Index: Low(~45)
Ingredients:
- 2 tuna steaks, 6 oz. each
- 1 avocado, peeled and sliced
- 2 C. mixed greens
- ½ red bell pepper, thinly sliced
- ¼ red onion, thinly sliced
- 1 lemon, juiced
- 2 Tbsp olive oil
- Salt and pepper to taste
- 1 tsp sesame seeds

Directions:
1. Season tuna steaks with salt and pepper
2. Heat olive oil in a pan over medium-high heat
3. Add tuna steaks and sear each side for 2 min
4. Remove from heat and slice thinly
5. In a large bowl, combine mixed greens, bell pepper, onion, avocado, and sliced tuna
6. Drizzle with lemon juice and toss gently
7. Sprinkle sesame seeds on top before serving

Tips:
- Opt for wild-caught tuna for better flavor and fewer contaminants

- Press sesame seeds into the tuna edges before searing for added texture and taste
- Squeeze extra lemon over your salad if you prefer a zesty flavor

Nutritional Values: Calories: 290, Fat: 15g, Carbs: 9g, Protein: 31g, Sugar: 2g, Sodium: 90mg, Potassium: 800mg, Cholesterol: 50mg

BEETROOT AND GOAT CHEESE ARUGULA SALAD

Preparation Time: 15 min
Cooking Time: none
Servings: 2
Glycemic Index: Low(~40)
Ingredients:
- 2 medium beetroots, cooked and sliced
- 1 C. arugula
- ½ C. goat cheese, crumbled
- ¼ C. walnuts, toasted
- 2 Tbsp balsamic vinegar
- 1 Tbsp extra-virgin olive oil
- Salt and pepper to taste

Directions:
1. Arrange arugula on a platter
2. Top with sliced beets and crumbled goat cheese
3. Sprinkle toasted walnuts over the salad
4. Drizzle with balsamic vinegar and olive oil
5. Season with salt and pepper to taste before serving

Tips:
- Consider roasting beetroots with a splash of olive oil for added depth of flavor
- Add orange slices for a sweet, tangy contrast
- Use pine nuts instead of walnuts for a different texture

Nutritional Values: Calories: 210, Fat: 15g, Carbs: 13g, Protein: 8g, Sugar: 9g, Sodium: 180mg, Potassium: 400mg, Cholesterol: 20mg

CUCUMBER AND FENNEL CITRUS SALAD

Preparation Time: 15 min
Cooking Time: none
Servings: 2
Glycemic Index: Low(~35)
Ingredients:
- 1 large cucumber, thinly sliced
- 1 small fennel bulb, thinly sliced
- 2 oranges, segmented
- 2 Tbsp olive oil
- 1 Tbsp white wine vinegar
- 1 tsp honey
- Salt and pepper to taste
- 2 Tbsp fennel fronds, chopped

Directions:
1. In a large bowl, combine cucumber, fennel bulb, and orange segments
2. In a small bowl, whisk together olive oil, white wine vinegar, honey, salt, and pepper
3. Pour dressing over the salad and toss to coat evenly
4. Garnish with fennel fronds before serving

Tips:
- Use a mandoline for evenly thin cucumber and fennel slices
- Replace honey with agave syrup if preferred
- Add toasted almonds for a crunchy texture

Nutritional Values: Calories: 160, Fat: 10g, Carbs: 18g, Protein: 2g, Sugar: 14g, Sodium: 20mg, Potassium: 430mg, Cholesterol: 0mg

BROCCOLI AND CHEDDAR SOUP

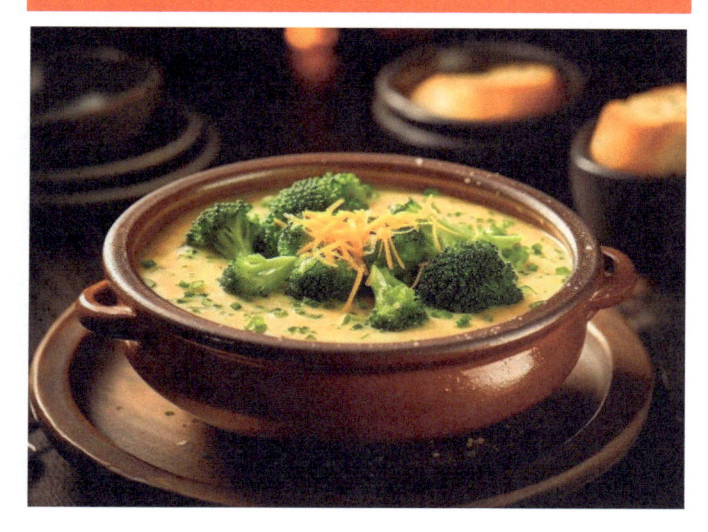

Preparation Time: 10 min
Cooking Time: 25 min
Servings: 4
Glycemic Index: Low(~50)
Ingredients:
- 2 Tbsp olive oil
- 1 onion, finely chopped
- 2 cloves garlic, minced
- 4 cups broccoli florets
- 3 cups vegetable broth
- 1 cup heavy cream
- 1 cup cheddar cheese, shredded
- ½ tsp nutmeg, ground
- Salt and pepper to taste

Directions:
1. Heat olive oil in a large pot over medium heat
2. Add chopped onion and minced garlic, sauté until translucent
3. Add broccoli florets and stir for 2 min
4. Pour in vegetable broth and bring to a boil, then reduce heat to simmer for 20 min
5. Blend until smooth using an immersion blender
6. Stir in heavy cream and cheddar cheese until cheese melts and soup is creamy
7. Season with nutmeg, salt, and pepper

Tips:
- Opt for low-sodium vegetable broth to further reduce sodium content
- Gradually add cheese to avoid clumping
- Serve with a sprinkle of extra cheddar for enhanced flavor

Nutritional Values: Calories: 290, Fat: 24g, Carbs: 10g, Protein: 9g, Sugar: 4g, Sodium: 410mg, Potassium: 350mg, Cholesterol: 90mg

TOMATO BASIL SOUP

Preparation Time: 5 min
Cooking Time: 30 min
Servings: 4
Glycemic Index: Low(~40)
Ingredients:
- 1 Tbsp olive oil
- 2 garlic cloves, minced
- 1 onion, diced
- 4 cups canned San Marzano tomatoes
- 2 cups low-sodium vegetable stock
- ½ cup basil leaves, fresh
- 1 Tbsp balsamic vinegar
- Salt and pepper to taste
- 1 tsp dried oregano

Directions:
1. Heat olive oil in a saucepan over medium heat
2. Add minced garlic and diced onion, cooking until onion becomes translucent
3. Add canned tomatoes, low-sodium vegetable stock, and oregano, bring to a simmer and cook for 25 min
4. Remove from heat, add fresh basil leaves and balsamic vinegar
5. Puree the soup with an immersion blender until smooth
6. Season with salt and pepper to taste

Tips:
- Use fresh basil for a more vibrant flavor
- Drizzle a bit of extra virgin olive oil before serving for a gourmet touch
- Add a dollop of low-fat Greek yogurt for creaminess without the fat

Nutritional Values: Calories: 90, Fat: 3g, Carbs: 14g, Protein: 3g, Sugar: 8g, Sodium: 190mg, Potassium: 290mg, Cholesterol: 0mg

Tempeh and Kale Pesto Wrap

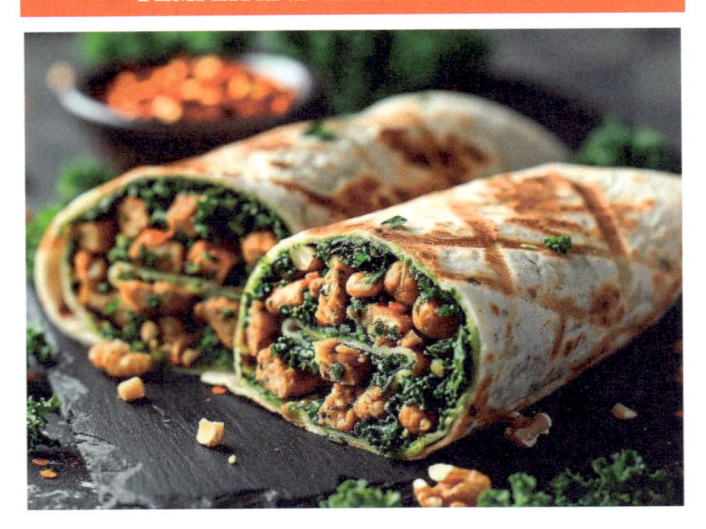

Preparation Time: 10 min
Cooking Time: 5 min
Servings: 2
Glycemic Index: Low(~48)
Ingredients:

- 2 Tbsp olive oil
- 4 oz tempeh, sliced
- 2 C. kale, de-stemmed and chopped
- ½ C. basil leaves
- 1 clove garlic
- 3 Tbsp walnuts
- 2 Tbsp nutritional yeast
- 1 lemon, juiced
- Salt and pepper to taste
- 4 whole grain tortilla wraps

Directions:

1. Preheat a sauté pan with olive oil and brown tempeh slices for about 2 minutes each side
2. In a food processor, blend kale, basil, garlic, walnuts, nutritional yeast, lemon juice, salt, and pepper until smooth to make pesto
3. Spread pesto on each tortilla, add tempeh slices, roll up the wraps tightly
4. Serve immediately or grill for 2-3 min for a crispy texture

Tips:

- Consider grilling the wrap to add crunchiness
- Swap walnuts with almonds for a different nutty flavor
- Enhance the pesto with a pinch of chili flakes for a spicy kick

Nutritional Values: Calories: 320, Fat: 15g, Carbs: 29g, Protein: 15g, Sugar: 3g, Sodium: 250mg, Potassium: 400mg, Cholesterol: 0mg

Spicy Pumpkin Soup

Preparation Time: 15 min
Cooking Time: 45 min
Servings: 4
Glycemic Index: Low(~55)
Ingredients:

- 1 medium pumpkin, peeled and cubed
- 1 Tbsp coconut oil
- 1 onion, chopped
- 3 cloves garlic, minced
- 1 Tbsp ginger, grated
- 4 cups vegetable broth
- 1 tsp cumin
- 1 tsp coriander
- ½ tsp cayenne pepper
- Salt and black pepper to taste
- ½ cup light coconut milk

Directions:

1. Toss cubed pumpkin with coconut oil and roast in the oven at 400°F (200°C) for 25 min
2. In a pot, sauté onion, garlic, and ginger until onion is soft
3. Add roasted pumpkin, vegetable broth, cumin, coriander, and cayenne pepper
4. Simmer for 20 min
5. Blend the mixture until smooth with an immersion blender
6. Stir in light coconut milk and season with salt and pepper

Tips:

- Choose light coconut milk for fewer calories and less fat
- Garnish with pumpkin seeds for added texture and a nutty flavor
- Incorporate a swirl of low-fat sour cream to balance the heat for those sensitive to spice

Nutritional Values: Calories: 180, Fat: 9g, Carbs: 23g, Protein: 3g, Sugar: 5g, Sodium: 300mg, Potassium: 500mg, Cholesterol: 0mg

QUINOA & BLACK BEAN SALAD JARS

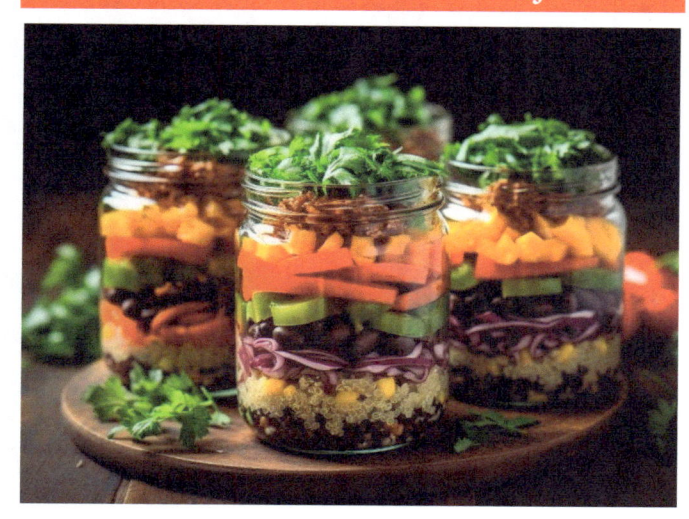

Preparation Time: 20 min
Cooking Time: none
Servings: 4
Glycemic Index: Low(~40)
Ingredients:

- 1 C. quinoa, cooked and cooled
- 1 C. black beans, rinsed and drained
- 1 red bell pepper, diced
- 1 C. cucumber, chopped
- 1/2 C. red onion, minced
- 1/4 C. parsley, chopped
- 3 Tbsp olive oil
- 2 Tbsp lemon juice
- 1 tsp ground cumin
- Salt and pepper to taste

Directions:

1. Layer ingredients in four medium-sized jars starting with quinoa, then black beans, red bell pepper, cucumber, and red onion
2. Top each jar with parsley, drizzle with olive oil and lemon juice, and sprinkle cumin, salt, and pepper
3. Seal the jars and refrigerate until ready to serve

Tips:

- Shake the jar before eating to mix the flavors
- If desired, top with crumbled feta cheese or avocado slices for extra richness
- Can be stored in the refrigerator for up to 4 days

Nutritional Values: Calories: 330, Fat: 10g, Carbs: 45g, Protein: 12g, Sugar: 3g, Sodium: 30mg, Potassium: 400mg, Cholesterol: 0mg

SMOKED CHICKEN CAESAR LETTUCE WRAP

Preparation Time: 15 min
Cooking Time: 10 min
Servings: 2
Glycemic Index: Low(~52)
Ingredients:

- 6 oz chicken breast, smoked and thinly sliced
- 1 C. Romaine lettuce, chopped
- ½ C. Parmesan cheese, shredded
- 2 Tbsp Greek yogurt
- 1 Tbsp Dijon mustard
- 1 tsp Worcestershire sauce
- 1 clove garlic, minced
- 1 Tbsp lemon juice
- 6 large lettuce leaves
- Salt and pepper to taste

Directions:

1. Mix Greek yogurt, Dijon mustard, Worcestershire sauce, garlic, lemon juice, salt, and pepper in a bowl to create dressing
2. Grill smoked chicken slices until just warmed through
3. Toss chicken, Romaine, and Parmesan with dressing
4. Spoon mixture into lettuce leaves, wrap tightly
5. Serve chilled or at room temperature

Tips:

- Use turkey as a lighter alternative to chicken
- Add anchovies to the dressing for a deeper umami flavor
- Prep these wraps in advance for a quick lunch option

Nutritional Values: Calories: 280, Fat: 16g, Carbs: 8g, Protein: 29g, Sugar: 2g, Sodium: 420mg, Potassium: 340mg, Cholesterol: 75mg

Sardine and Chickpea Salad Pita

Preparation Time: 12 min
Cooking Time: none
Servings: 2
Glycemic Index: Medium(~65)
Ingredients:
- 1 can sardines in olive oil, drained
- 1 C. chickpeas, rinsed and drained
- ¼ C. red onion, finely chopped
- 1 small cucumber, diced
- 2 Tbsp parsley, chopped
- 2 Tbsp lemon juice
- 1 tsp paprika
- 4 whole wheat pita pockets
- Salt and pepper to taste

Directions:
1. In a large bowl, combine sardines, chickpeas, red onion, cucumber, parsley, lemon juice, paprika, salt, and pepper
2. Evenly distribute the salad among the pita pockets, gently filling them

Tips:
- Add a drizzle of extra virgin olive oil for extra richness
- Sprinkle a bit of feta cheese for a Mediterranean touch
- Use roasted red peppers instead of paprika for a smoky flavor

Nutritional Values: Calories: 310, Fat: 12g, Carbs: 34g, Protein: 20g, Sugar: 4g, Sodium: 580mg, Potassium: 480mg, Cholesterol: 45mg

Chicken and Walnut Pesto Wraps

Preparation Time: 15 min
Cooking Time: none
Servings: 6
Glycemic Index: Low(~40)
Ingredients:
- 6 whole wheat tortillas
- 2 C. cooked chicken, shredded
- 1/2 C. carrots, julienned
- 1/2 C. zucchini, julienned
- 1/4 C. walnuts, chopped
- 1/4 C. basil leaves, fresh
- 3 Tbsp olive oil
- 2 cloves garlic, minced
- 2 Tbsp parmesan cheese, grated
- Salt and pepper to taste

Directions:
1. Prepare pesto by blending walnuts, basil leaves, olive oil, garlic, parmesan, salt, and pepper until smooth
2. Spread pesto on tortillas
3. Top with shredded chicken, carrots, and zucchini
4. Roll tortillas tightly and cut in half before serving

Tips:
- Store leftover pesto in a sealed container in the fridge
- Use spinach instead of basil for a different flavor profile
- Add sundried tomatoes for extra zest

Nutritional Values: Calories: 295, Fat: 13g, Carbs: 27g, Protein: 20g, Sugar: 2g, Sodium: 210mg, Potassium: 180mg, Cholesterol: 30mg

Mediterranean Tuna and Barley Salad

Preparation Time: 25 min
Cooking Time: none
Servings: 4
Glycemic Index: Medium(~65)
Ingredients:
- 1 C. barley, cooked and cooled
- 2 cans tuna in water, drained
- 1/2 C. cherry tomatoes, halved
- 1/4 C. Kalamata olives, pitted and halved
- 1/2 C. artichoke hearts, quartered
- 1/4 C. feta cheese, crumbled
- 3 Tbsp olive oil
- 2 Tbsp red wine vinegar
- 1 tsp dried oregano
- Salt and pepper to taste

Directions:
1. In a large mixing bowl, combine barley, tuna, cherry tomatoes, olives, and artichoke hearts

2. Add olive oil, red wine vinegar, and dried oregano
3. Season with salt and pepper
4. Toss well to combine all the ingredients
5. Sprinkle with feta cheese before serving

Tips:
- Serve chilled or at room temperature
- For a gluten-free option, replace barley with cooked quinoa
- Add cucumber and red onions for more crunch and flavor

Nutritional Values: Calories: 350, Fat: 18g, Carbs: 32g, Protein: 20g, Sugar: 3g, Sodium: 320mg, Potassium: 270mg, Cholesterol: 25mg

DINNER

Dinner—the meal that placates our daily hunger and brings families together as the sun dips below the horizon. But when you're managing diabetes, particularly in the golden years beyond 50, dinner is not just a meal but a crucial part of your health regimen. Let's reframe the way we view this evening staple: it's not about what you can't eat, but how what you eat can enhance your life.

Imagine settling in for an evening meal that satisfies not just your tastebuds but also supports your health challenges and goals. With the right recipes and knowledge at your disposal, a delicious, low-carb, and low-sugar dinner can be both a reality and a delight. By incorporating wholesome ingredients with robust flavors, your dinner plate can showcase a rainbow of nutrients that help manage blood sugar levels, protect heart health, and stave off other diabetes-related complications.

At this point, some might worry about the complexity and time involved in preparing such nutritious meals. However, the recipes captured here honor your time and your palate. They are crafted to be straightforward, ensuring that even those new to the kitchen can feel empowered to cook. From savory slow-cooked stews that simmer while you savor the peace of your afternoon to vibrant salads that assemble in minutes, each recipe is designed to minimize kitchen time and maximize flavor and health benefits.

And as we include every family member in our mealtime rituals, these dishes also cater to all palates, ensuring that adhering to a diabetic-friendly diet doesn't mean dining in solitude. You can prepare a single meal that everyone at the table can enjoy, making those shared moments around the dinner table as nourishing for the heart as they are for the body.

So, as we dive into this chapter, remember that each recipe is more than just a set of instructions; it's a gateway to enriching your health and your life through the joy of flavorful, wholesome food that aligns with your dietary needs. Let's transform your evening meal into a powerful tool in your diabetes management arsenal, one delicious bite at a time.

ZUCCHINI RIBBON AND TURKEY BACON SKILLET

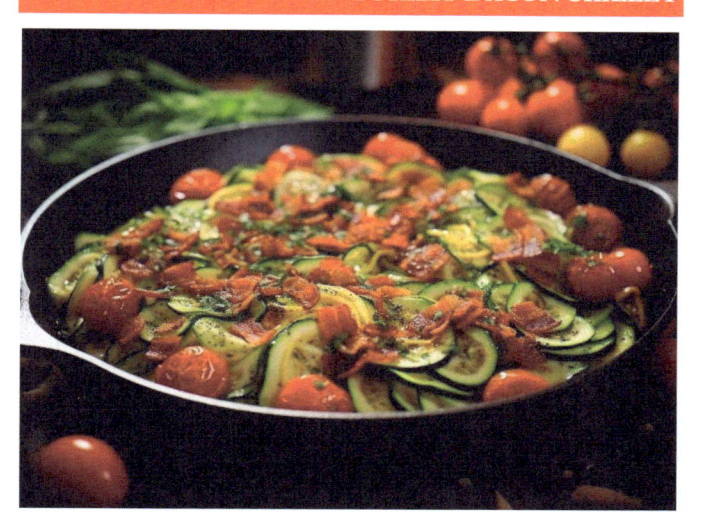

Preparation Time: 15 min
Cooking Time: 20 min
Servings: 4
Glycemic Index: Low(~35)
Ingredients:

- 2 large zucchini, thinly sliced into ribbons
- 8 slices turkey bacon, chopped
- 1 medium onion, finely diced
- 2 cloves garlic, minced
- 1 cup cherry tomatoes, halved
- ¼ cup fresh basil, chopped
- 1 Tbsp olive oil
- Salt and pepper to taste

Directions:

1. Heat olive oil in a large skillet over medium heat
2. Add turkey bacon and cook until crisp, about 5-7 min
3. Add onion and garlic, sauté until onion is translucent, about 5 min
4. Add zucchini ribbons and cherry tomatoes, cook until zucchini is tender but still firm, about 3-4 min
5. Season with salt and pepper

6. Garnish with fresh basil before serving

Tips:
- Pair with a sprinkle of grated Parmesan for enhanced flavor
- Opt for smoked turkey bacon for a deeper taste
- Serve alongside a portion of quinoa for added fiber

Nutritional Values: Calories: 210, Fat: 12g, Carbs: 10g, Protein: 14g, Sugar: 4g, Sodium: 480mg, Potassium: 340mg, Cholesterol: 30mg

LEMON HERB ROASTED CHICKEN THIGHS

Preparation Time: 10 min
Cooking Time: 45 min
Servings: 4
Glycemic Index: Low(~40)
Ingredients:
- 4 chicken thighs, bone-in and skin-on
- 1 lemon, sliced
- 2 Tbsp fresh rosemary, chopped
- 2 Tbsp fresh thyme, chopped
- 4 cloves garlic, minced
- 2 Tbsp olive oil
- Salt and pepper to taste
- 1 tsp paprika

Directions:
1. Preheat oven to 375°F (190°C)
2. Arrange chicken thighs in a roasting tray
3. Drizzle with olive oil and rub with garlic, rosemary, thyme, paprika, salt, and pepper
4. Place lemon slices around and under the chicken
5. Roast in the oven until the skin is crispy and the chicken is cooked through, about 45 min

Tips:
- Utilize fresh herbs for a more potent flavor
- Squeeze roasted lemon over chicken before serving for extra zest
- Serve with steamed green beans for a complete meal

Nutritional Values: Calories: 280, Fat: 22g, Carbs: 3g, Protein: 19g, Sugar: 1g, Sodium: 420mg, Potassium: 230mg, Cholesterol: 80mg

GRILLED TOFU AND ASPARAGUS WITH TAHINI SAUCE

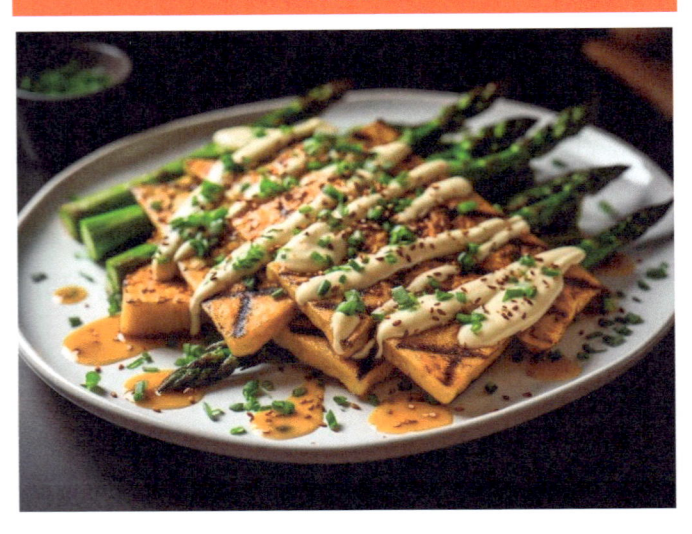

Preparation Time: 15 min
Cooking Time: 10 min
Servings: 2
Glycemic Index: Low(~40)
Ingredients:
- 14 oz. firm tofu, pressed and sliced
- 1 lb. asparagus, trimmed
- 1 Tbsp olive oil
- Salt to taste
- 2 Tbsp tahini
- 1 Tbsp lemon juice
- 1 clove garlic, minced
- 1 tsp maple syrup
- 3 Tbsp water

Directions:
1. Press tofu to remove excess moisture and slice into 1/2 inch pieces
2. Brush tofu and asparagus with olive oil and lightly season with salt
3. Grill tofu and asparagus over medium heat, turning occasionally, until tofu is golden and asparagus is tender, about 10 min
4. For sauce, whisk together tahini, lemon juice, minced garlic, maple syrup, and water until smooth
5. Drizzle sauce over grilled tofu and asparagus before serving

Tips:
- Serve with a sprinkle of sesame seeds for extra crunch and flavor
- Adjust the amount of water in sauce for desired consistency
- Grill lemon halves alongside for a smoky citrus garnish

Nutritional Values: Calories: 280, Fat: 19g, Carbs: 18g, Protein: 19g, Sugar: 5g, Sodium: 200mg, Potassium: 512mg, Cholesterol: 0mg

SPICED CAULIFLOWER STEAKS WITH TURMERIC AND CUMIN

Preparation Time: 10 min
Cooking Time: 30 min
Servings: 2
Glycemic Index: Low(~45)
Ingredients:
- 1 large head of cauliflower, sliced into 1-inch thick steaks
- 1 Tbsp olive oil
- 1 tsp turmeric powder
- 1 tsp cumin seeds
- ½ tsp salt
- ½ tsp black pepper
- 2 Tbsp cilantro, chopped for garnish

Directions:
1. Preheat oven to 400°F (204°C)
2. Brush cauliflower steaks with olive oil and sprinkle with turmeric, cumin seeds, salt, and pepper
3. Lay on a baking sheet and bake until golden and tender, about 25-30 min
4. Garnish with cilantro before serving

Tips:
- Introduce a squeeze of lemon for a refreshing taste
- Pair with a side of mint yogurt sauce to complement the spices
- Ensure steaks are not overcrowded on the baking sheet for even roasting

Nutritional Values: Calories: 110, Fat: 7g, Carbs: 10g, Protein: 4g, Sugar: 3g, Sodium: 300mg, Potassium: 430mg, Cholesterol: 0mg

ZESTY LEMON GARLIC TILAPIA

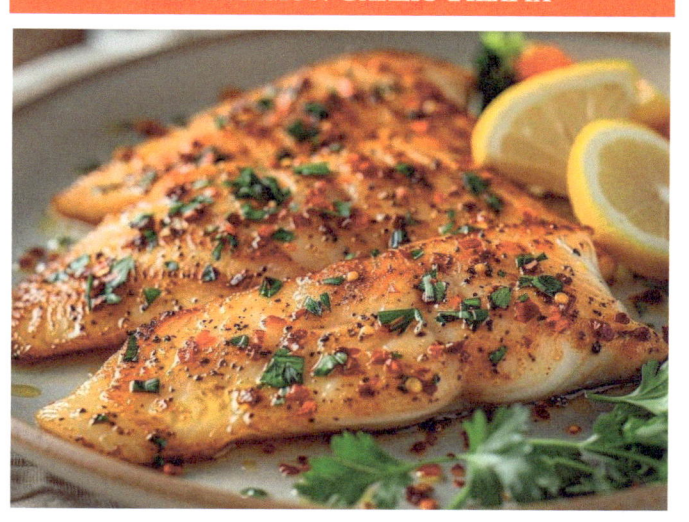

Preparation Time: 15 min
Cooking Time: 20 min
Servings: 4
Glycemic Index: Medium(~59)
Ingredients:
- 4 tilapia fillets, 6 oz. each
- 3 Tbsp olive oil
- 2 cloves garlic, minced
- 1 lemon, zest and juice
- 1 Tbsp parsley, chopped
- ½ tsp paprika
- ¼ tsp black pepper
- 1 tsp dried oregano

Directions:
1. Preheat oven to 375°F (190°C)
2. In a small bowl, combine olive oil, garlic, lemon zest and juice, parsley, paprika, black pepper, and oregano to make the marinade
3. Place tilapia fillets in a baking dish and cover evenly with the marinade
4. Let sit for 10 min, then bake in the oven for 20 min or until fish flakes easily with a fork

Tips:
- To ensure even cooking, position fillets in a single layer in the baking dish

- For a crispier top, broil for the last 2-3 min of cooking
- Serve with a side of steamed vegetables for a complete meal

Nutritional Values: Calories: 200, Fat: 10g, Carbs: 2g, Protein: 28g, Sugar: 1g, Sodium: 70mg, Potassium: 450mg, Cholesterol: 60mg

CAULIFLOWER STEAKS WITH ROMESCO SAUCE

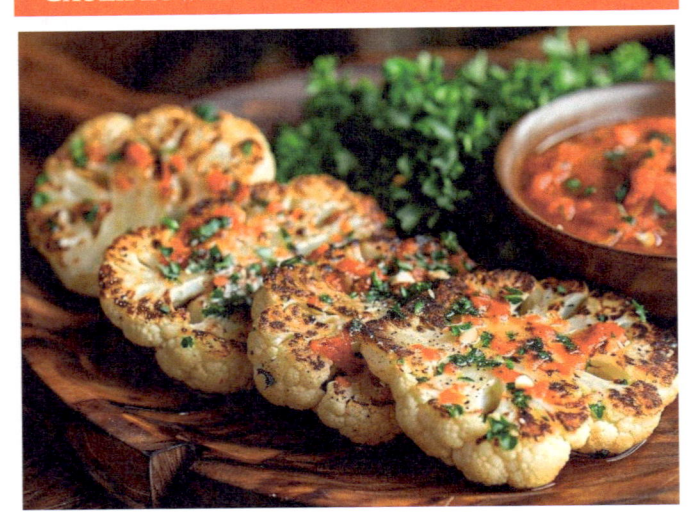

Preparation Time: 10 min
Cooking Time: 25 min
Servings: 2
Glycemic Index: Low(~45)

Ingredients:
- 1 large head cauliflower, sliced into steaks
- 1 cup roasted red peppers, drained
- 1/4 cup almonds, toasted
- 2 cloves garlic
- 2 Tbsp sherry vinegar
- 2 Tbsp olive oil
- 1/2 tsp smoked paprika
- Salt and pepper to taste

Directions:
1. Preheat oven to 400°F (200°C)
2. Arrange cauliflower steaks on a baking sheet and brush with 1 Tbsp olive oil, season with salt and pepper
3. Roast until tender and browned, about 25 min
4. For the romesco, blend roasted red peppers, almonds, garlic, sherry vinegar, 1 Tbsp olive oil, smoked paprika in a food processor until smooth

Tips:
- Pair with a green salad to add a fresh contrast
- Store leftover romesco sauce in fridge to enhance flavors for use in other dishes
- Add a pinch of cayenne to romesco for additional heat

Nutritional Values: Calories: 210, Fat: 15g, Carbs: 16g, Protein: 6g, Sugar: 6g, Sodium: 300mg, Potassium: 860mg, Cholesterol: 0mg

ZUCCHINI RIBBON SALAD WITH LEMON AND HERBS

Preparation Time: 20 min
Cooking Time: none
Servings: 2
Glycemic Index: Low(~35)

Ingredients:
- 3 medium zucchini, thinly sliced lengthwise
- 1 Tbsp extra virgin olive oil
- 2 Tbsp lemon juice
- 1 tsp lemon zest
- 1/4 cup fresh basil, chopped
- 1/4 cup fresh mint, chopped
- Salt and pepper to taste
- 1/4 cup pine nuts, toasted

Directions:
1. Use a vegetable peeler to slice zucchini into thin ribbons
2. In a large bowl, whisk together olive oil, lemon juice, lemon zest
3. Add zucchini, basil, and mint to the bowl and toss gently to coat
4. Season with salt and pepper and sprinkle with toasted pine nuts before serving

Tips:
- Serve immediately to preserve the crispness of the zucchini
- If desired, incorporate crumbled feta for a salty kick
- Increase lemon zest for a brighter flavor

Nutritional Values: Calories: 150, Fat: 12g, Carbs: 10g, Protein: 4g, Sugar: 4g, Sodium: 80mg, Potassium: 450mg, Cholesterol: 0mg

Slow-Cooked Mediterranean Chicken

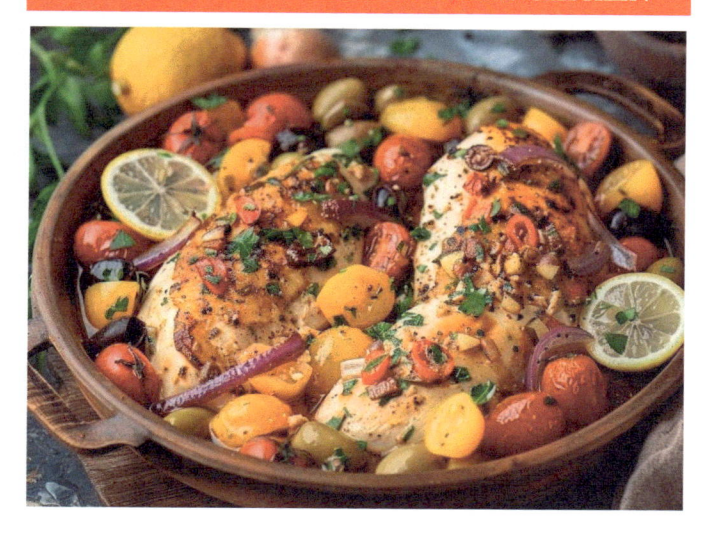

Preparation Time: 10 min
Cooking Time: 4 hr
Servings: 4
Glycemic Index: Low(~40)
Ingredients:

- 4 boneless, skinless chicken breasts
- 1 C. cherry tomatoes, halved
- 1 yellow bell pepper, sliced
- 1 red onion, quartered
- 3 cloves garlic, minced
- ¼ C. kalamata olives, pitted
- 1 lemon, sliced
- 2 Tbsp olive oil
- 1 tsp dried oregano
- ½ tsp salt
- ¼ tsp black pepper
- ¼ C. feta cheese, crumbled
- 2 Tbsp fresh parsley, chopped

Directions:

1. Place chicken breasts at the bottom of the slow cooker
2. Top with cherry tomatoes, bell pepper, red onion, garlic, and kalamata olives
3. Arrange lemon slices over the top
4. Drizzle olive oil and sprinkle oregano, salt, and pepper
5. Cover and cook on low for 4 hr
6. Garnish with feta cheese and fresh parsley before serving

Tips:

- To enhance the flavors, sear chicken breasts lightly before placing in the slow cooker
- Replace kalamata olives with capers for a tangier taste
- Serve with a side of quinoa for a complete meal

Nutritional Values: Calories: 310, Fat: 15g, Carbs: 12g, Protein: 32g, Sugar: 3g, Sodium: 485mg, Potassium: 570mg, Cholesterol: 85mg

Stuffed Bell Peppers with Quinoa and Turkey

Preparation Time: 20 min
Cooking Time: 30 min
Servings: 4
Glycemic Index: Medium(~65)
Ingredients:

- 4 large bell peppers, tops cut and seeded
- 1 lb ground turkey, 93% lean
- 1 cup quinoa, cooked
- 1 onion, finely chopped
- 2 cloves garlic, minced
- 1 cup crushed tomatoes
- 1 tsp cumin
- ½ tsp chili flakes
- ¼ cup cilantro, chopped
- 2 Tbsp olive oil

Directions:

1. Preheat oven to 350°F (177°C)
2. In a skillet, heat olive oil and sauté onion and garlic until translucent
3. Add ground turkey and cook until browned
4. Stir in quinoa, crushed tomatoes, cumin, chili flakes, and half the cilantro, cooking for an additional 5 min
5. Stuff the prepared bell peppers with the turkey quinoa mixture and place them in a baking dish
6. Bake for 30 min or until peppers are tender

Tips:

- Serve with a dollop of Greek yogurt on top for extra creaminess
- For a spicier kick, increase the amount of chili flakes

- Garnish with remaining cilantro before serving

Nutritional Values: Calories: 360, Fat: 16g, Carbs: 35g, Protein: 24g, Sugar: 7g, Sodium: 180mg, Potassium: 670mg, Cholesterol: 80mg

HERB CRUSTED SALMON WITH FENNEL SALAD

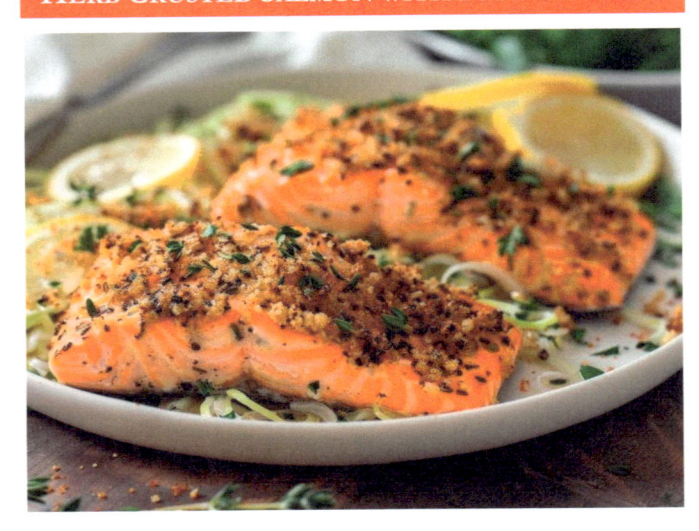

Preparation Time: 10 min
Cooking Time: 15 min
Servings: 4
Glycemic Index: Low(~45)
Ingredients:

- 4 salmon fillets, 4 oz. each
- 2 Tbsp Dijon mustard
- ½ cup whole wheat breadcrumbs
- 1 Tbsp thyme, freshly chopped
- 1 Tbsp rosemary, freshly chopped
- 1 fennel bulb, thinly sliced
- 2 Tbsp olive oil
- 1 lemon, juice only
- Salt and pepper to taste

Directions:

1. Preheat oven to 400°F (204°C)
2. Spread Dijon mustard on each salmon fillet
3. In a bowl, mix breadcrumbs, thyme, and rosemary, then press onto the mustard-coated fillets
4. Place fillets on a greased baking sheet and bake for 15 min
5. For the salad, toss fennel slices in a bowl with olive oil, lemon juice, salt, and pepper

Tips:

- Avoid overcooking the salmon to maintain its moisture and tenderness
- Pair the fennel salad with a vinaigrette for added flavor
- Use panko breadcrumbs for a crunchier crust

Nutritional Values: Calories: 290, Fat: 15g, Carbs: 10g, Protein: 27g, Sugar: 3g, Sodium: 200mg, Potassium: 550mg, Cholesterol: 75mg

TUSCAN PORK TENDERLOIN

Preparation Time: 15 min
Cooking Time: 6 hr
Servings: 6
Glycemic Index: Low(~45)
Ingredients:

- 2 lb pork tenderloin
- 1 C. diced tomatoes, canned
- 1 C. baby spinach
- ½ C. low-sodium chicken broth
- 1 C. mushrooms, sliced
- 1 Tbsp Italian seasoning
- 2 cloves garlic, minced
- 1 tsp salt
- ½ tsp black pepper
- ¼ C. freshly grated Parmesan cheese

Directions:

1. Place pork tenderloin into the slow cooker
2. Top with diced tomatoes, baby spinach, mushrooms, and garlic
3. Pour chicken broth over the ingredients
4. Season with Italian seasoning, salt, and black pepper
5. Cover and cook on low for 6 hr
6. Sprinkle with Parmesan cheese before serving

Tips:

- Thinly slice the cooked pork for a more refined presentation
- Baby arugula can substitute for spinach for a sharper flavor
- Enjoy this dish with a glass of dry red wine to complement the Tuscan flavors

Nutritional Values: Calories: 295, Fat: 10g, Carbs: 6g, Protein: 42g, Sugar: 2g, Sodium: 640mg, Potassium: 950mg, Cholesterol: 110mg

ONE-PAN SALMON WITH ASPARAGUS

Preparation Time: 5 min
Cooking Time: 25 min
Servings: 4
Glycemic Index: Low(~50)
Ingredients:

- 4 salmon fillets, 6 oz each
- 1 lb asparagus, trimmed
- 1 lemon, sliced
- 2 Tbsp olive oil
- 1 tsp garlic powder
- 1 tsp dried dill
- ½ tsp salt
- ¼ tsp black pepper

Directions:

1. Preheat oven to 400°F (200°C)
2. Arrange salmon fillets and asparagus on a single baking sheet
3. Drizzle with olive oil and sprinkle garlic powder, dill, salt, and black pepper
4. Top with lemon slices
5. Bake in the oven for 25 min or until salmon is cooked through

Tips:

- Line the baking sheet with parchment paper for easier cleanup
- Squeeze extra lemon juice over the salmon right after baking for added zest
- Pair with a chilled white wine like Sauvignon Blanc to enhance the dining experience

Nutritional Values: Calories: 345, Fat: 21g, Carbs: 5g, Protein: 34g, Sugar: 2g, Sodium: 350mg, Potassium: 810mg, Cholesterol: 90mg

SNACKS AND SIDES

Navigating the dietary waters of diabetes after 50 can feel like sailing against the tide, especially when it comes to finding suitable snacks and sides that are both delightful and diet-compliant. It's often in these smaller meals where sugar and carbs sneak their way into our daily routine, disguised in the most innocuous snacks. Yet, it is here, in the realm of the seemingly trivial, where we can make impactful decisions that significantly boost our diabetic management.

Imagine laying out a table for a family gathering or preparing a quick mid-afternoon treat for yourself. The challenge isn't just in the preparation but in choosing ingredients that harmonize with your health needs without compromising flavor. Many fear that adapting to a diabetes-friendly diet means bidding adieu to enjoyable snacks and sides. But what if I told you that it's a myth we're about to debunk together?

In this chapter, we journey through a selection of snacks and side dishes designed not just to satisfy your cravings but to stabilize your blood sugar levels and nourish your body. From zesty, roasted vegetables that transform a mundane Tuesday dinner into a celebration, to innovative, low-carb finger foods that promise to be the highlights of your next social gathering, each recipe is crafted keeping you in mind.

We dive into flavors from different cultures, weaving in herbs and spices known for their health benefits, integrating them into your diet in the most delicious ways. Think of cinnamon that not only tickles your taste buds but also aids in reducing your blood sugar levels, or turmeric that brings its anti-inflammatory prowess to your meals.

Let's embrace the art of crafting snacks and sides that are as nutritious as they are enticing. With each recipe, you'll find not just a set of instructions but a gateway to an enriched lifestyle, proving that every small dish can contribute to a larger canvas of health and vigor. Engage your senses, invite curiosity, and let's make our snack times a testament to our dedication to health, without ever feeling deprived.

ROASTED CHICKPEA AND KALE POPPERS

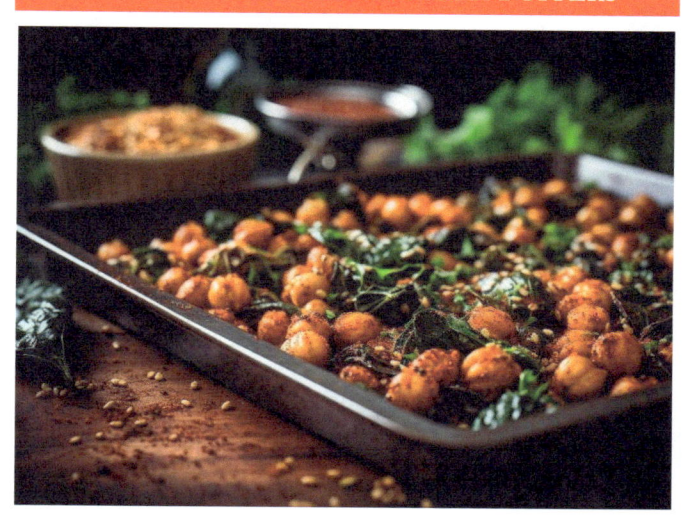

Preparation Time: 10 min
Cooking Time: 25 min
Servings: 4
Glycemic Index: Low(~48)
Ingredients:
- 1 can (15 oz.) chickpeas, rinsed and drained
- 2 cups kale, finely chopped
- 1 Tbsp olive oil
- ½ tsp smoked paprika
- ¼ tsp garlic powder
- ¼ tsp onion powder
- Salt and pepper to taste

Directions:
1. Preheat oven to 400°F (200°C)
2. Pat chickpeas dry with a paper towel and remove any loose skins
3. In a bowl, combine chickpeas, chopped kale, olive oil, smoked paprika, garlic powder, onion powder, salt, and pepper, and mix until well coated
4. Spread the mixture evenly on a baking sheet
5. Bake for 25 min., stirring halfway through, until chickpeas are golden and crispy

Tips:
- Spread the kale in a single layer to ensure it crisps up
- Add a pinch of cayenne pepper for extra spice
- Serve warm for best texture and flavor

Nutritional Values: Calories: 150, Fat: 6g, Carbs: 20g, Protein: 6g, Sugar: 4g, Sodium: 300mg, Potassium: 275mg, Cholesterol: 0mg

ZUCCHINI BASIL BITES

Preparation Time: 15 min
Cooking Time: none
Servings: 2
Glycemic Index: Low(~43)

Ingredients:
- 1 large zucchini, grated
- 1 egg, beaten
- ¼ cup almond flour
- 2 Tbsp basil, fresh, minced
- 1 small clove garlic, minced
- 2 Tbsp Parmesan cheese, grated
- Salt and pepper to taste
- 1 Tbsp olive oil for greasing

Directions:
1. Grate zucchini and squeeze out excess liquid with a clean cloth
2. In a large bowl, combine grated zucchini, beaten egg, almond flour, minced basil, minced garlic, grated Parmesan, salt, and pepper, and mix well to form a consistent batter
3. Grease a mini muffin pan with olive oil
4. Spoon the zucchini mixture into the muffin cups
5. Refrigerate for 10 min. to set
6. Serve chilled or at room temperature

Tips:
- Chill before serving to enhance flavors and firm up the bites
- Pair with a side of marinara sauce for dipping
- Use fresh basil for a more vibrant flavor

Nutritional Values: Calories: 80, Fat: 5g, Carbs: 4g, Protein: 4g, Sugar: 2g, Sodium: 125mg, Potassium: 200mg, Cholesterol: 30mg

ROASTED RED PEPPER AND WALNUT DIP

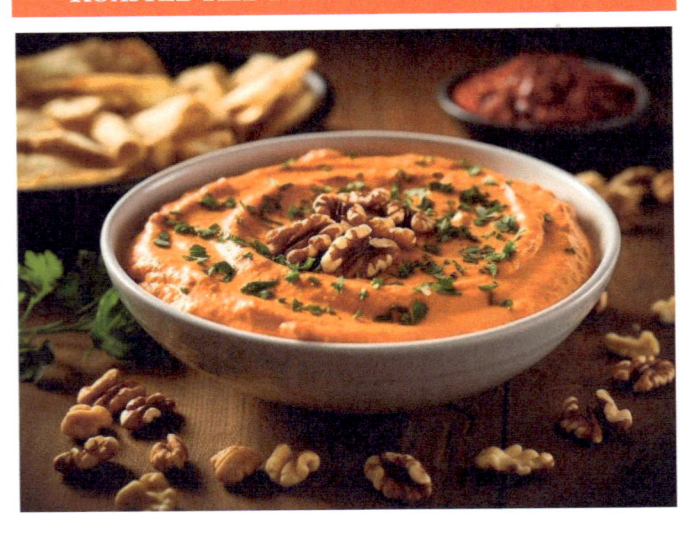

Preparation Time: 10 min
Cooking Time: none
Servings: 4
Glycemic Index: Low(~35)

Ingredients:
- 1 C. roasted red peppers, drained
- ½ C. walnuts, toasted
- 2 Tbsp olive oil
- 1 garlic clove, minced
- 1 Tbsp lemon juice
- ¼ tsp smoked paprika
- ¼ tsp cumin
- Salt and pepper to taste

Directions:
1. Combine roasted red peppers, walnuts, olive oil, minced garlic, lemon juice, smoked paprika, and cumin in a blender
2. Blend until smooth
3. Season with salt and pepper to taste
4. Transfer to a serving dish and chill before serving

Tips:
- Add a sprinkle of chopped parsley for a fresh garnish
- Blend on high for a smoother texture
- Store in an airtight container, refrigerated, for up to 4 days

Nutritional Values: Calories: 140, Fat: 13g, Carbs: 4g, Protein: 2g, Sugar: 2g, Sodium: 240mg, Potassium: 95mg, Cholesterol: 0mg

Cucumber Roll-Ups with Feta and Sun-dried Tomatoes

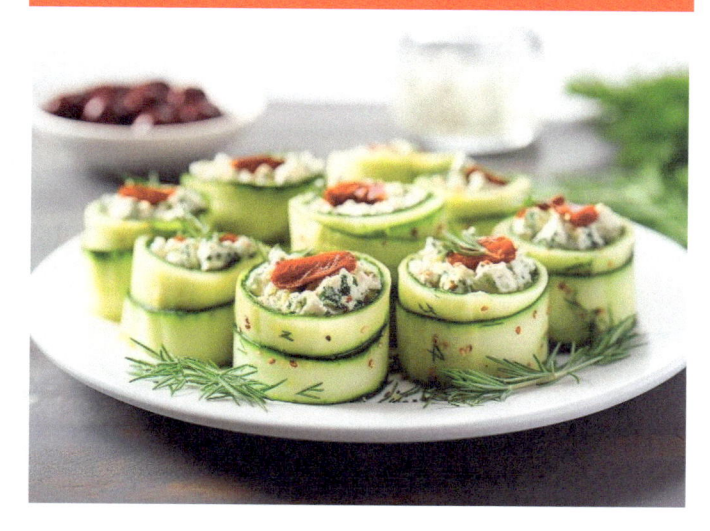

Preparation Time: 20 min
Cooking Time: none
Servings: 6
Glycemic Index: Low(~45)
Ingredients:

- 1 large cucumber
- ½ cup feta cheese, crumbled
- ¼ cup sun-dried tomatoes, chopped
- 2 Tbsp Kalamata olives, pitted and chopped
- 1 Tbsp dill, chopped
- 1 Tbsp lemon juice
- Salt and pepper to taste

Directions:

1. Peel cucumber and slice lengthwise into thin strips using a mandoline slicer
2. In a small bowl, mix crumbled feta cheese, chopped sun-dried tomatoes, chopped olives, chopped dill, and lemon juice, and season with salt and pepper to taste
3. Lay cucumber strips flat and spoon a small amount of the feta mixture onto one end of each strip
4. Roll up tightly and secure with a toothpick

Tips:

- Serve immediately or chill briefly to meld flavors
- Opt for oil-packed sun-dried tomatoes for extra richness
- Remove toothpicks before serving if preferred

Nutritional Values: Calories: 60, Fat: 4g, Carbs: 3g, Protein: 2g, Sugar: 2g, Sodium: 400mg, Potassium: 125mg, Cholesterol: 5mg

Herbed Ricotta and Chive Spread

Preparation Time: 15 min
Cooking Time: none
Servings: 3
Glycemic Index: Low(~50)
Ingredients:

- 1 C. ricotta cheese, part-skim
- 2 Tbsp chives, chopped
- 1 Tbsp parsley, fresh, chopped
- 1 tsp lemon zest
- Salt and black pepper to taste
- Dash of nutmeg

Directions:

1. In a medium bowl, mix together ricotta cheese, chives, parsley, and lemon zest
2. Season with salt, pepper, and a dash of nutmeg
3. Mix until all ingredients are well incorporated
4. Refrigerate for about 1 hr before serving to allow flavors to blend

Tips:

- Serve with vegetable sticks or low-carb crackers for a satisfying snack
- Use whole-milk ricotta for a creamier texture if desired
- Add a pinch of chili flakes for a spicy kick

Nutritional Values: Calories: 90, Fat: 5g, Carbs: 3g, Protein: 7g, Sugar: 2g, Sodium: 80mg, Potassium: 120mg, Cholesterol: 20mg

Spicy Pumpkin Seed Dip

Preparation Time: 8 min
Cooking Time: none
Servings: 4
Glycemic Index: Low(~45)
Ingredients:

- 1 C. pumpkin seeds, roasted and unsalted

- 1 small jalapeño, seeded and chopped
- ½ C. cilantro leaves
- 2 Tbsp lime juice
- 1 Tbsp olive oil
- 1 tsp honey
- ¼ tsp salt

Directions:
1. Place pumpkin seeds, jalapeño, cilantro, lime juice, olive oil, and honey in a food processor
2. Process until the mixture is smooth and creamy
3. Season with salt
4. Transfer to a bowl and serve chilled or at room temperature

Tips:
- For a less spicy version, reduce the jalapeño by half
- Drizzle with a bit of extra virgin olive oil before serving for added richness
- Can be stored in the refrigerator for up to 5 days in an airtight container

Nutritional Values: Calories: 158, Fat: 13g, Carbs: 5g, Protein: 7g, Sugar: 1g, Sodium: 150mg, Potassium: 129mg, Cholesterol: 0mg

Spicy Bok Choy in Garlic Sauce

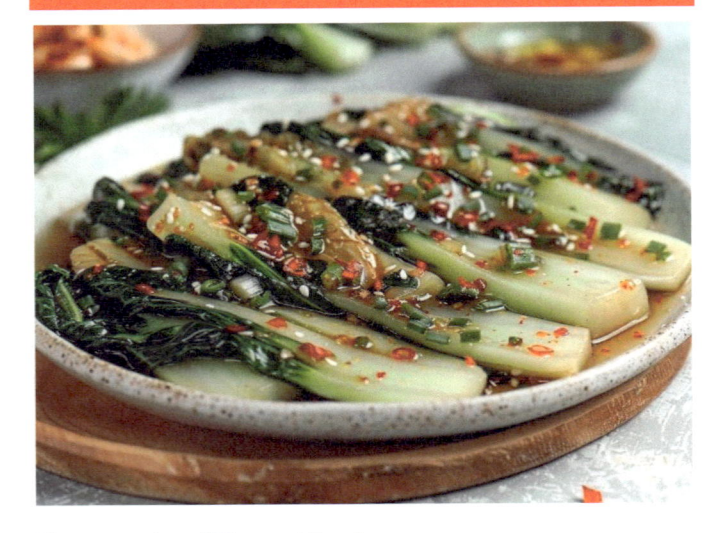

Preparation Time: 10 min
Cooking Time: 5 min
Servings: 4
Glycemic Index: Low(~35)
Ingredients:
- 2 lb. bok choy, cleaned and chopped
- 4 cloves garlic, minced
- 1 Tbsp ginger, freshly grated
- 2 Tbsp low-sodium soy sauce
- 1 Tbsp olive oil
- 1 tsp chili flakes
- 1 Tbsp sesame seeds
- ½ tsp black pepper, ground

Directions:
1. Heat olive oil in a large skillet over medium heat
2. Add garlic and ginger, sauté until aromatic, about 1 min
3. Add bok choy, soy sauce, chili flakes, and black pepper to the skillet
4. Cook, stirring occasionally, until bok choy is tender but crisp, about 4 min
5. Garnish with sesame seeds before serving

Tips:
- Add a splash of sesame oil for an extra nutty flavor
- Adjust chili flakes according to heat preference
- Serve alongside grilled fish or chicken for a balanced meal

Nutritional Values: Calories: 60, Fat: 3.5g, Carbs: 4.5g, Protein: 2.5g, Sugar: 1.5g, Sodium: 230mg, Potassium: 530mg, Cholesterol: 0mg

Roasted Acorn Squash with Herbs and Pecans

Preparation Time: 15 min
Cooking Time: 25 min
Servings: 4
Glycemic Index: Low(~55)
Ingredients:
- 1 acorn squash, halved and seeded
- 1 Tbsp olive oil
- 2 tsp rosemary, fresh, minced
- 2 tsp thyme, fresh, minced
- ¼ C. pecans, chopped
- Salt to taste
- Black pepper, ground, to taste

Directions:
1. Preheat oven to 375°F (190°C)

2. Brush acorn squash halves with olive oil and season with salt and pepper
3. Sprinkle rosemary and thyme evenly over the squash
4. Place on a baking sheet cut side up and roast until tender, about 25 min
5. Sprinkle roasted squash with chopped pecans before serving

Tips:
- Choose smaller acorn squash for sweeter flavor
- Add a drizzle of maple syrup for a subtle sweetness if desired
- Pecans can be substituted with walnuts for a different texture

Nutritional Values: Calories: 145, Fat: 9g, Carbs: 16g, Protein: 2g, Sugar: 3g, Sodium: 10mg, Potassium: 487mg, Cholesterol: 0mg

CAULIFLOWER TABBOULEH

Preparation Time: 20 min
Cooking Time: none
Servings: 6
Glycemic Index: Low(~45)
Ingredients:
- 1 head cauliflower, riced
- 1 C. parsley, finely chopped
- 1/2 C. mint, finely chopped
- 2 tomatoes, diced
- 1 cucumber, diced
- 3 Tbsp olive oil
- Juice of 1 lemon
- Salt to taste
- Black pepper, ground, to taste

Directions:
1. In a large mixing bowl, combine riced cauliflower, parsley, mint, tomatoes, and cucumber
2. Add olive oil and lemon juice, season with salt and pepper to taste
3. Mix thoroughly to combine all ingredients
4. Chill in the refrigerator before serving to enhance flavors

Tips:
- Use a food processor to rice the cauliflower for a finer texture
- Lemon zest can be added for an extra citrus kick
- Serve as a refreshing side with grilled chicken or lamb

Nutritional Values: Calories: 77, Fat: 5g, Carbs: 7g, Protein: 2g, Sugar: 3g, Sodium: 30mg, Potassium: 430mg, Cholesterol: 0mg

ROSEMARY-SPICED NUTS

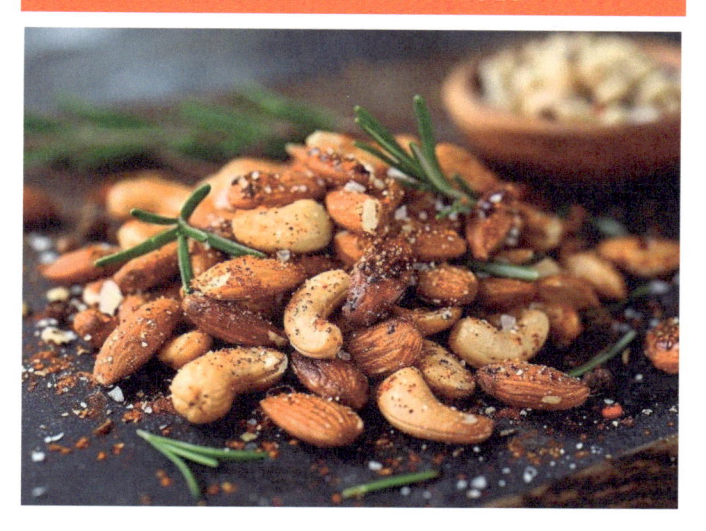

Preparation Time: 10 min
Cooking Time: 15 min
Servings: 4
Glycemic Index: Low(~15)
Ingredients:
- 1 C. almonds
- 1 C. walnuts
- 1 Tbsp extra virgin olive oil
- 2 tsp dried rosemary
- ¼ tsp cayenne pepper
- ½ tsp garlic powder
- Salt to taste

Directions:
1. Preheat oven to 350°F (175°C)
2. In a bowl, mix almonds and walnuts with olive oil, rosemary, cayenne pepper, garlic powder, and salt
3. Spread the nuts on a baking sheet in a single layer

4. Bake for 15 min, stirring halfway through to ensure even roasting
5. Remove from oven and let cool before serving

Tips:
- Store in an airtight container to maintain freshness
- Add a sprinkle of smoked paprika for an extra kick of flavor
- Experiment with different nuts like pecans or hazelnuts for variety

Nutritional Values: Calories: 210, Fat: 20g, Carbs: 6g, Protein: 6g, Sugar: 1g, Sodium: 90mg, Potassium: 200mg, Cholesterol: 0mg

CHILLED CUCUMBER CUPS

Preparation Time: 15 min
Cooking Time: none
Servings: 6
Glycemic Index: Low(~28)

Ingredients:
- 3 large cucumbers, cut into 2-inch slices
- 1 C. cottage cheese, low-fat
- 1 Tbsp dill, finely chopped
- 1 tsp lemon juice
- Salt and pepper to taste
- ½ tsp chili flakes

Directions:
1. Hollow out the center of each cucumber slice to form a cup
2. In a bowl, combine cottage cheese, dill, lemon juice, salt, and pepper
3. Spoon the cottage cheese mixture into each cucumber cup
4. Sprinkle chili flakes on top for a spicy finish
5. Serve chilled

Tips:
- For a creamy texture, blend the cottage cheese before filling the cups
- Use lime juice instead of lemon for a tangy twist
- Decorate with a sprig of mint for additional freshness

Nutritional Values: Calories: 50, Fat: 1.5g, Carbs: 4g, Protein: 4g, Sugar: 2g, Sodium: 200mg, Potassium: 150mg, Cholesterol: 5mg

SMOKED SALMON & CREAM CHEESE PINWHEELS

Preparation Time: 20 min
Cooking Time: none
Servings: 12
Glycemic Index: Low(~30)

Ingredients:
- 6 oz smoked salmon, thinly sliced
- 4 oz cream cheese, low-fat
- 4 whole wheat tortillas
- 1 Tbsp capers
- ½ C. arugula
- 1 tsp lemon zest
- Salt and pepper to taste

Directions:
1. Lay a tortilla flat and spread an even layer of cream cheese over it
2. Top with smoked salmon, capers, arugula, and lemon zest
3. Season with salt and pepper
4. Carefully roll the tortilla tightly into a log
5. Slice the log into 1-inch thick pinwheels
6. Serve immediately or chill before serving

Tips:
- Use flavored cream cheese for extra taste
- Place toothpicks in each pinwheel before chilling to maintain their shape
- Serve with a side of Greek yogurt dip for added flavor

Nutritional Values: Calories: 70, Fat: 3g, Carbs: 5g, Protein: 5g, Sugar: 1g, Sodium: 230mg, Potassium: 60mg, Cholesterol: 10mg

Diabetic-Friendly Desserts

The end of a meal often brings with it the anticipation of a sweet finale. Desserts hold a beloved spot in many cultures and family traditions, serving not just as a treat but as a gesture of hospitality and celebration. For those managing diabetes particularly past the age of 50, indulging in dessert might seem like a challenge steeped in guilt and complications. How does one revel in the pleasure of sweets while keeping blood sugar under control?

In this chapter, we delve into the art of crafting diabetic-friendly desserts that excite the palate without spiking your glucose levels. Imagine the warmth of cinnamon-spiced baked apples, the smoothness of a chocolate avocado mousse, or the refreshing zest of a berry parfait. These aren't merely substitution-based versions of traditional desserts; they are reimagined, health-conscious treats designed to delight while respecting your body's needs.

Creating desserts that are both low in carbohydrates and sugars and high in flavor and texture requires an understanding of ingredients and their interactions. Think of almond flour's nutty essence tenderly embracing the moistness in cakes, or the natural sweetness of ripe berries reducing the need for added sugars. Here, the beauty lies not just in enjoying what you eat, but also in knowing that what you're eating supports your health journey.

Moreover, the shared experience of dessert should not be understated. It's a common concern—how to partake in social gatherings without the worry of dietary restrictions overshadowing the joy of the moment. The recipes featured in this chapter not only meet your dietary needs but are also appealing and satisfying for all your loved ones, regardless of their health conditions. This way, you can stay connected in those precious social settings without feeling isolated or anxious about your food choices.

Desserts, in the context of a diabetic diet, are not just about indulgence but also innovation, inclusion, and intimacy. Let's rediscover the joy of desserts through a lens that is both healthful and heartwarming, crafting moments of sweetness that contribute to your well-being without compromise.

Almond Flour Lemon Bars

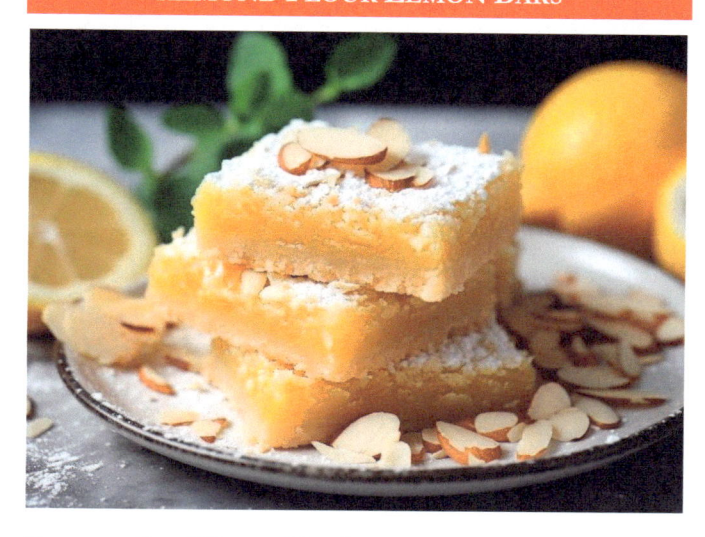

Preparation Time: 20 min
Cooking Time: 25 min
Servings: 12
Glycemic Index: Low(~35)
Ingredients:

- 2 cups almond flour
- ⅓ cup coconut oil, melted
- 2 Tbsp stevia
- 1 pinch salt
- 3 large eggs
- 1 cup fresh lemon juice
- 1 Tbsp lemon zest
- ¼ cup stevia
- 2 Tbsp coconut flour

Directions:

1. Combine almond flour, coconut oil, 2 Tbsp stevia, and salt in a bowl and mix until crumbly
2. Press the mixture into the bottom of a lightly greased 9x9 inch baking pan and bake at 350°F (175°C) for 15 min
3. Whisk eggs, lemon juice, lemon zest, ¼ cup stevia, and coconut flour in a bowl until smooth
4. Pour over the baked crust and return to the oven for an additional 25 min
5. Cool completely before cutting into bars

Tips:
- Use parchment paper for easy removal of bars from the pan
- Refrigerate bars before serving to enhance the flavors and texture
- Serve with a sprinkle of powdered erythritol for extra sweetness without impacting glycemic load

Nutritional Values: Calories: 190, Fat: 15g, Carbs: 8g, Protein: 6g, Sugar: 1g, Sodium: 45mg, Potassium: 35mg, Cholesterol: 55mg

COCONUT CHIA PUDDING

Preparation Time: 10 min
Cooking Time: none
Servings: 4
Glycemic Index: Low(~30)
Ingredients:
- 1 can coconut milk, full-fat
- ¼ cup chia seeds
- 1 Tbsp stevia
- 1 tsp vanilla extract
- 1 pinch cinnamon

Directions:
1. Mix coconut milk, chia seeds, stevia, vanilla extract, and cinnamon in a bowl until well combined
2. Cover and refrigerate overnight to allow chia seeds to swell and thicken the mixture
3. Stir well before serving and add extra toppings like berries or nuts if desired

Tips:
- Add a splash of almond milk for a thinner consistency if preferred
- Top with unsweetened toasted coconut flakes for added texture and flavor
- Enhance sweetness naturally with a few drops of stevia if desired

Nutritional Values: Calories: 280, Fat: 25g, Carbs: 12g, Protein: 4g, Sugar: 1g, Sodium: 15mg, Potassium: 200mg, Cholesterol: 0mg

ALMOND FLOUR LEMON CAKE

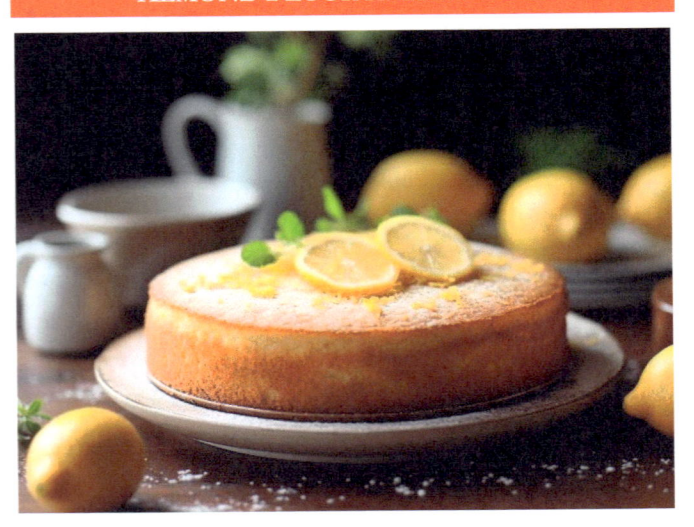

Preparation Time: 15 min
Cooking Time: 30 min
Servings: 8
Glycemic Index: Low(~35)
Ingredients:
- 2½ C. almond flour
- ½ C. erythritol
- 1 tsp baking powder
- ¼ tsp salt
- 4 eggs, large
- ¼ C. olive oil
- ½ C. unsweetened almond milk
- 2 Tbsp lemon zest
- ¼ C. lemon juice
- 1 tsp vanilla extract

Directions:
1. Preheat oven to 350°F (175°C)
2. In a large bowl, mix almond flour, erythritol, baking powder, and salt
3. In another bowl, whisk eggs, olive oil, almond milk, lemon zest, lemon juice, and vanilla extract
4. Combine wet and dry ingredients and stir until smooth
5. Pour batter into a greased 9-inch cake pan
6. Bake for 30 min or until a toothpick inserted into the center comes out clean
7. Let cool before serving

Tips:
- Use fresh lemon zest for the best flavor

- A dollop of unsweetened whipped cream can enhance the serving presentation
- Store cake in an airtight container to keep it moist

Nutritional Values: Calories: 280, Fat: 23g, Carbs: 10g, Protein: 8g, Sugar: 2g, Sodium: 120mg, Potassium: 50mg, Cholesterol: 85mg

ALMOND BUTTER CHOCOLATE ENERGY BALLS

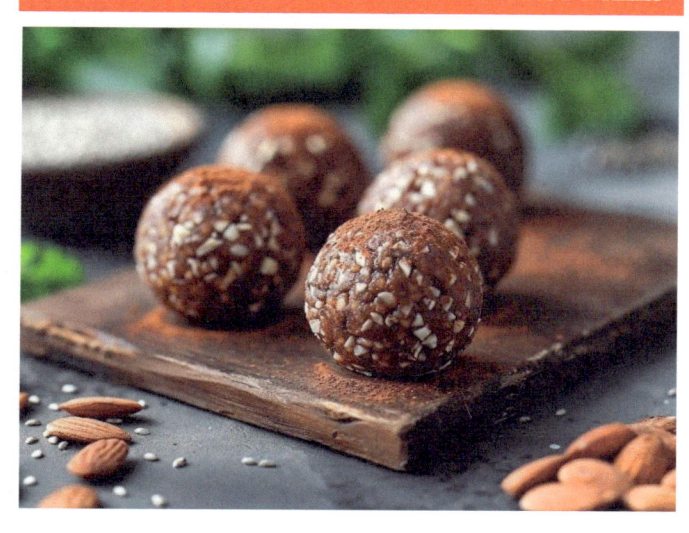

Preparation Time: 20 min
Cooking Time: none
Servings: 10
Glycemic Index: Low(~40)
Ingredients:
- 1 C. almond butter, unsweetened
- 2 Tbsp cocoa powder, unsweetened
- ½ C. flaxseed meal
- ¼ C. hemp seeds
- 2 Tbsp coconut oil
- ¼ tsp salt
- 1 tsp cinnamon

Directions:
1. In a mixing bowl, blend almond butter, cocoa powder, flaxseed meal, hemp seeds, coconut oil, salt, and cinnamon until well combined
2. Roll the mixture into small balls, each about an inch in diameter
3. Chill in the refrigerator for 15 minutes to set

Tips:
- Store in an airtight container in the fridge for easy snack access throughout the week
- Add a sprinkle of chia seeds for extra nutrients and texture
- Swap hemp seeds for pumpkin seeds for a variation in flavor

Nutritional Values: Calories: 100, Fat: 8g, Carbs: 4g, Protein: 3g, Sugar: 1g, Sodium: 25mg, Potassium: 95mg, Cholesterol: 0mg

SPICED BAKED PEAR HALVES

Preparation Time: 10 min
Cooking Time: 30 min
Servings: 4
Glycemic Index: Low(~40)
Ingredients:
- 2 large pears, halved and cored
- 1 Tbsp butter, unsalted
- 2 Tbsp erythritol
- 1 tsp ground cinnamon
- ¼ tsp ground nutmeg
- ¼ tsp ground cloves
- 1 Tbsp chopped pecans

Directions:
1. Place the pear halves on a baking sheet with cut sides up and dot each with butter
2. Mix erythritol, cinnamon, nutmeg, and cloves together and sprinkle over the pears
3. Bake in a preheated oven at 375°F (190°C) for 30 min or until the pears are tender
4. Garnish with chopped pecans before serving

Tips:
- Serve warm with a dollop of unsweetened whipped cream for extra indulgence
- Experiment with different spices like cardamom or ginger for a unique flavor twist
- Pears can be pre-baked and reheated to save time during busy times

Nutritional Values: Calories: 120, Fat: 4g, Carbs: 21g, Protein: 1g, Sugar: 14g, Sodium: 5mg, Potassium: 85mg, Cholesterol: 10mg

Pumpkin Spice Muffins with Stevia

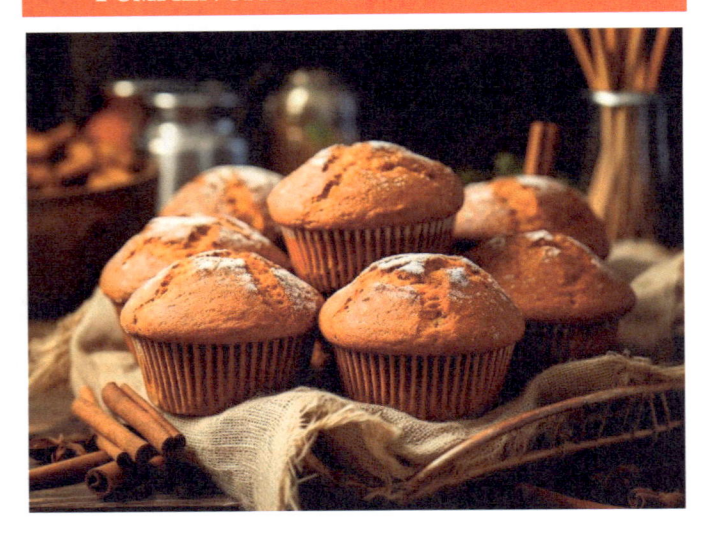

Preparation Time: 20 min
Cooking Time: 25 min
Servings: 12
Glycemic Index: Medium(~60)
Ingredients:
- 1¾ C. whole wheat flour
- 1 tsp baking soda
- ¼ tsp salt
- 1 tsp ground cinnamon
- ½ tsp ground ginger
- ¼ tsp ground nutmeg
- ¼ tsp ground cloves
- 1 C. pumpkin puree
- ⅓ C. melted coconut oil
- ½ C. stevia
- ¼ C. water
- 1 tsp vanilla extract

Directions:
1. Preheat oven to 375°F (190°C)
2. In a bowl, combine whole wheat flour, baking soda, salt, cinnamon, ginger, nutmeg, and cloves
3. In another bowl, mix pumpkin puree, melted coconut oil, stevia, water, and vanilla extract
4. Add the wet ingredients to the dry ingredients and mix just until combined
5. Spoon the batter into prepared muffin tins, filling each cup about ¾ full
6. Bake for 25 min or until a toothpick comes out clean
7. Allow muffins to cool on a wire rack

Tips:
- Opt for organic pumpkin puree for a richer taste and pesticide-free option
- Incorporate a handful of walnuts for added texture and nutrients
- Muffins stay fresh longer when stored in a cool, dry place

Nutritional Values: Calories: 150, Fat: 9g, Carbs: 16g, Protein: 3g, Sugar: 1g, Sodium: 210mg, Potassium: 80mg, Cholesterol: 0mg

Coconut Flour Chocolate Chip Cookies

Preparation Time: 10 min
Cooking Time: 15 min
Servings: 15
Glycemic Index: Low(~40)
Ingredients:
- 1¼ C. coconut flour
- ½ C. erythritol
- ¼ tsp salt
- ½ tsp baking powder
- ½ C. butter, softened
- 2 eggs
- 1 tsp vanilla extract
- ¼ C. unsweetened almond milk
- ½ C. sugar-free chocolate chips

Directions:
1. Preheat oven to 375°F (190°C)
2. In a large bowl, mix coconut flour, erythritol, salt, and baking powder
3. Add softened butter, eggs, vanilla extract, and almond milk to the dry ingredients and mix until a dough forms
4. Fold in the sugar-free chocolate chips
5. Drop tablespoons of dough onto a baking sheet lined with parchment paper
6. Bake for 15 min until edges are golden brown
7. Transfer to a wire rack to cool

Tips:
- Experiment with adding chopped nuts for extra crunch and protein

- Keep cookies in a tightly sealed container to maintain freshness
- Mixing by hand rather than with an electric mixer can help avoid overmixing the dough

Nutritional Values: Calories: 130, Fat: 9g, Carbs: 9g, Protein: 3g, Sugar: 1g, Sodium: 95mg, Potassium: 15mg, Cholesterol: 30mg

GRILLED PEACH WITH RICOTTA AND BASIL

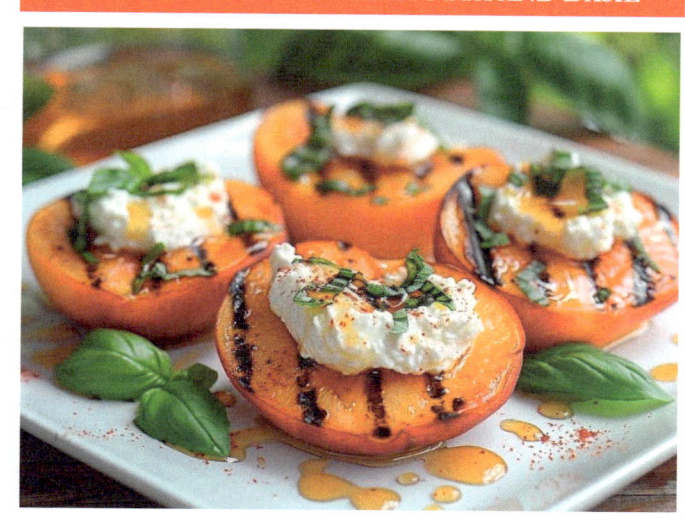

Preparation Time: 15 min
Cooking Time: 6 min
Servings: 4
Glycemic Index: Low(~45)
Ingredients:
- 4 peaches, halved and pitted
- 1 cup ricotta cheese
- 2 Tbsp honey
- ¼ cup basil leaves, freshly chopped
- 1 Tbsp olive oil
- A pinch of salt

Directions:
1. Preheat grill to medium-high heat (375°F/190°C)
2. Brush peach halves with olive oil and place on the grill cut side down
3. Grill for about 3 minutes each side or until they have nice grill marks and are slightly softened
4. Mix ricotta with honey and salt in a bowl
5. Place grilled peaches on plates, top each with a dollop of honey ricotta and sprinkle with freshly chopped basil leaves
6. Serve warm

Tips:
- Opt for part-skim ricotta to reduce fat content
- Drizzle additional honey if a sweeter touch is desired, but cautiously to keep sugar intake low
- Fresh mint can be a vibrant alternative to basil

Nutritional Values: Calories: 155, Fat: 8g, Carbs: 18g, Protein: 6g, Sugar: 16g, Sodium: 85mg, Potassium: 210mg, Cholesterol: 20mg

NO-BAKE LEMON CHEESECAKE CUPS

Preparation Time: 30 min
Cooking Time: none
Servings: 4
Glycemic Index: Low(~35)
Ingredients:
- 1 C. cashews, soaked overnight and drained
- ¼ C. lemon juice, fresh
- 2 tsp lemon zest
- ⅓ C. coconut oil, melted
- ¼ C. erythritol
- ½ tsp vanilla extract
- 1 C. raspberries for garnish

Directions:
1. Blend soaked cashews, lemon juice, lemon zest, melted coconut oil, erythritol, and vanilla extract in a blender until smooth and creamy
2. Divide the mixture evenly among four small bowls or cups
3. Refrigerate for at least an hour to set
4. Top each cup with fresh raspberries before serving

Tips:
- Opt for refrigerating overnight to fully enhance the flavors
- Garnish with a sprinkle of lemon zest for an extra zing
- Ensure all ingredients, especially the lemon juice, are fresh for best results

Nutritional Values: Calories: 280, Fat: 24g, Carbs: 10g, Protein: 6g, Sugar: 3g, Sodium: 5mg, Potassium: 200mg, Cholesterol: 0mg

Strawberry Rhubarb Compote with Mint

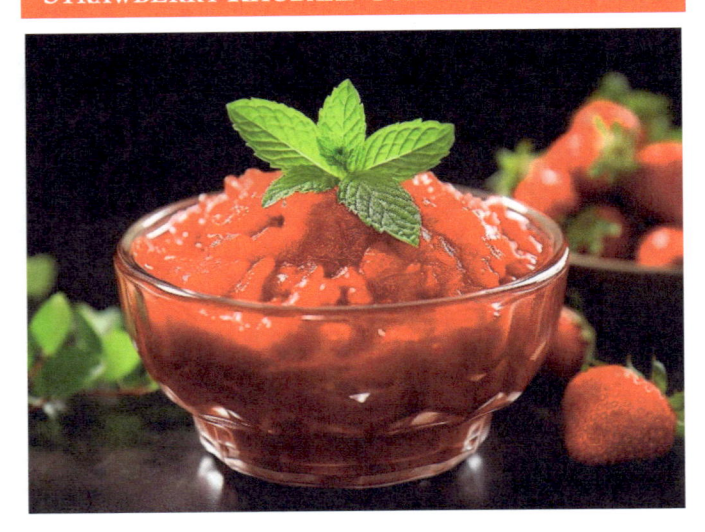

Preparation Time: 10 min
Cooking Time: 15 min
Servings: 4
Glycemic Index: Low(~30)
Ingredients:
- 2 cups rhubarb, diced
- 1 cup strawberries, sliced
- ¼ cup xylitol
- ½ cup water
- Juice of 1 lemon
- 1 Tbsp mint leaves, chopped

Directions:
1. Combine rhubarb, strawberries, xylitol, water, and lemon juice in a saucepan over medium heat
2. Bring to a boil, then reduce heat and let it simmer for about 15 minutes or until the fruit is tender and the compote has thickened
3. Remove from heat and stir in chopped mint leaves
4. Serve warm or chill in the refrigerator before serving

Tips:
- Sweeten further with stevia instead of sugar to keep it diabetes-friendly
- Serve over low-fat Greek yogurt for a nutritious dessert or breakfast option
- Prepare in large batches and store in the fridge for up to one week

Nutritional Values: Calories: 60, Fat: 0.5g, Carbs: 14g, Protein: 1g, Sugar: 5g, Sodium: 5mg, Potassium: 220mg, Cholesterol: 0mg

Pistachio and Date Bars

Preparation Time: 25 min
Cooking Time: none
Servings: 8
Glycemic Index: Low(~45)
Ingredients:
- 2 C. dates, pitted and roughly chopped
- 1 C. pistachios, shelled
- 1/2 C. coconut flakes, unsweetened
- 1/4 tsp salt
- 2 Tbsp coconut oil, melted
- 1 tsp orange zest

Directions:
1. Process dates, pistachios, coconut flakes, salt, melted coconut oil, and orange zest in a food processor until the mixture forms a sticky dough
2. Press the dough into a lined baking sheet, flattening to about half an inch thick
3. Freeze for 20 minutes, then cut into bars

Tips:
- These bars can be stored in the freezer for up to a month
- Wrap individually for a quick, portable snack
- Add a scoop of protein powder for an extra protein boost

Nutritional Values: Calories: 210, Fat: 12g, Carbs: 23g, Protein: 4g, Sugar: 18g, Sodium: 65mg, Potassium: 300mg, Cholesterol: 0mg

Blueberry Mango Chia Pudding

Preparation Time: 10 min
Cooking Time: none
Servings: 2
Glycemic Index: Low(~35)
Ingredients:
- 1 mango, peeled and diced
- ½ cup blueberries
- ¼ cup chia seeds

- 1 cup unsweetened almond milk
- 1 tsp vanilla extract
- 1 tbsp shredded coconut, unsweetened

Directions:

1. Combine chia seeds, almond milk, and vanilla extract in a bowl
2. Stir thoroughly to mix
3. Refrigerate for at least 4 hours or overnight until it reaches a pudding consistency
4. Once set, layer chia pudding with diced mango and blueberries in serving glasses
5. Top each serving with shredded coconut
6. Serve chilled

Tips:

- To enhance flavor, allow pudding to sit for an additional hour after adding fruits before serving
- Use coconut milk for a richer texture and tropical flavor
- Top with a sprinkle of cinnamon or nutmeg for added spice

Nutritional Values: Calories: 210, Fat: 10g, Carbs: 27g, Protein: 5g, Sugar: 15g, Sodium: 30mg, Potassium: 320mg, Cholesterol: 0mg

30 Days Meal Plan

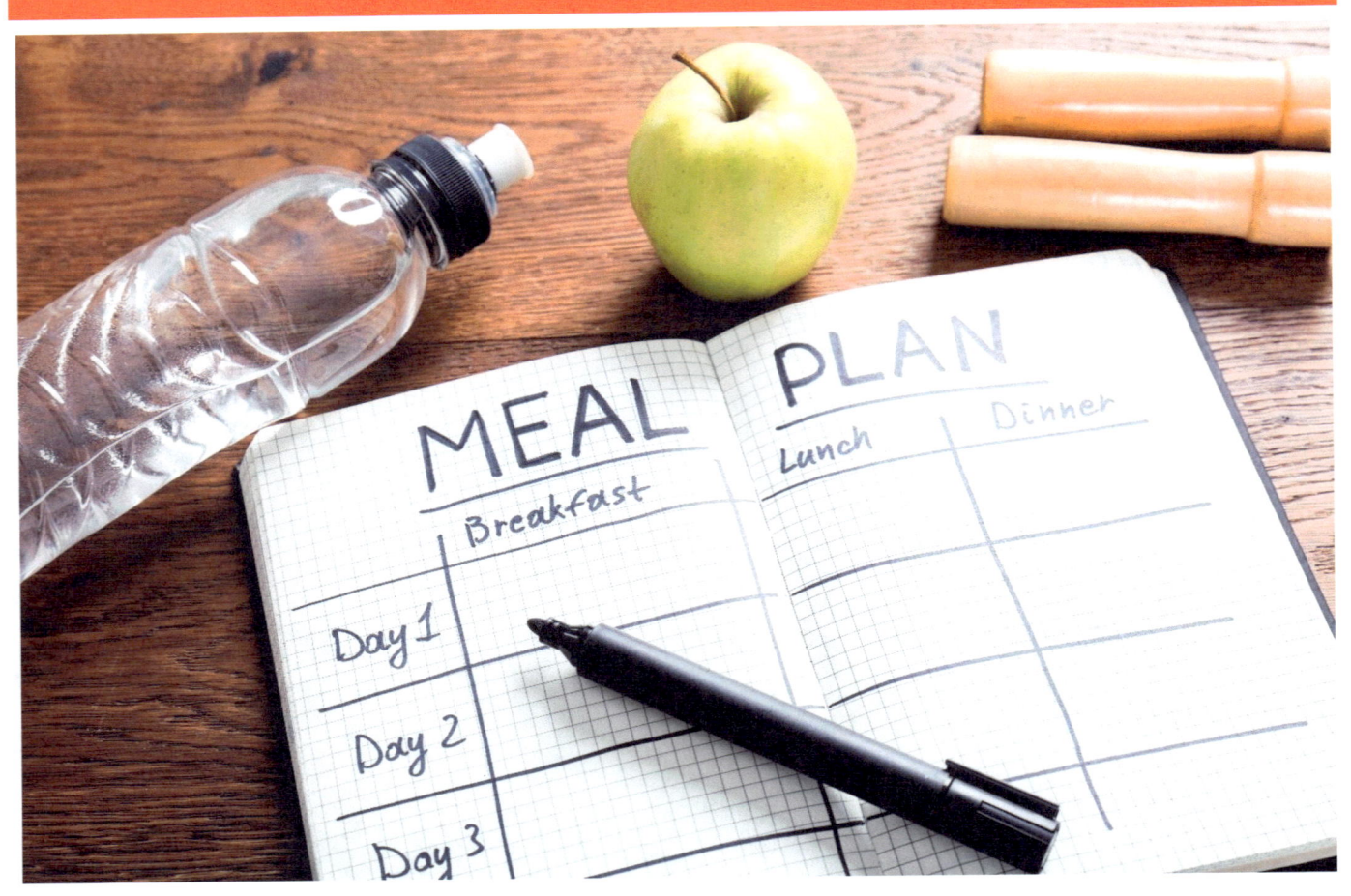

Embarking on a journey to manage diabetes after 50 can be as exciting as it is daunting. But imagine waking each morning with a clear plan—the right meals at the right times—not just any food, but delicious, nourishing dishes that leave you satisfied and energized. This is not just a dream; it's a reality within these pages of your 30-day meal plan.

Crafting this plan, I thought deeply about our common challenges and aspirations. Whether you're reeling from a recent diagnosis or have battled diabetes for years, the goal is universal: to enjoy our meals without fear and to nourish our bodies without compromise. Each recipe and each day's meal in this plan is a stepping stone to regaining control over your health. They ensure you're not just eating, but thriving.

Why a 30-day outline, you might ask? It's more than just a set period; it's about setting a habit. Psychologists say it takes about a month to establish new habits. Thus, this structured path is designed to help you integrate new eating patterns seamlessly into your life, long after these 30 days pass. It's structured enough to give you confidence, yet flexible enough to adjust to your pace and preferences.

From hearty breakfasts that power your morning without spiking your sugar levels, to sumptuous dinners that make you forget the word 'diet,' each recipe is your ally. And let's not overlook the joys of snacks—yes, snacks that you can love without guilt or worry, thoughtfully included to keep your energy up and your sugars down throughout the day.

As you turn these pages, picture the meals as more than food; see them as your partners in a vibrant, healthier life. This plan isn't just about managing diabetes; it's about reclaiming the joy of eating and living well. Let's step into this journey with optimism and a spoonful of enthusiasm, ready to enjoy every bite along the way.

	breakfast	snack	lunch	snack	dinner
Day 01	Broccoli and Feta Omelet	Roasted Chickpea and Kale Poppers	Seared Tuna and Avocado Salad	Almond Flour Lemon Bars	Zucchini Ribbon and Turkey Bacon Skillet
Day 02	Chia and Almond Yogurt Parfait	Zucchini Basil Bites	Beetroot and Goat Cheese Arugula Salad	Coconut Chia Pudding	Lemon Herb Roasted Chicken Thighs
Day 03	Spinach and Mushroom Egg Muffins	Cucumber Roll-Ups with Feta and Sun-dried Tomatoes	Cucumber and Fennel Citrus Salad	Spiced Baked Pear Halves	Spiced Cauliflower Steaks with Turmeric and Cumin
Day 04	Turmeric Tofu Scramble	Roasted Red Pepper and Walnut Dip	Broccoli and Cheddar Soup	Almond Flour Lemon Cake	Grilled Tofu and Asparagus with Tahini Sauce
Day 05	Chia and Hemp Seed Yogurt Parfait	Herbed Ricotta and Chive Spread	Tomato Basil Soup	Pumpkin Spice Muffins with Stevia	Cauliflower Steaks with Romesco Sauce
Day 06	Smoked Salmon and Avocado Tartine	Spicy Pumpkin Seed Dip	Spicy Pumpkin Soup	Coconut Flour Chocolate Chip Cookies	Zucchini Ribbon Salad with Lemon and Herbs
Day 07	Berry Ginger Zinger Smoothie	Spicy Bok Choy in Garlic Sauce	Tempeh and Kale Pesto Wrap	Almond Butter Chocolate Energy Balls	Zesty Lemon Garlic Tilapia
Day 08	Cucumber Melon Medley Shake	Roasted Acorn Squash with Herbs and Pecans	Smoked Chicken Caesar Lettuce Wrap	No-Bake Lemon Cheesecake Cups	Stuffed Bell Peppers with Quinoa and Turkey
Day 09	Peaches and Cream Oat Shake	Cauliflower Tabbouleh	Sardine and Chickpea Salad Pita	Pistachio and Date Bars	Herb Crusted Salmon with Fennel Salad
Day 10	Chia and Coconut Yogurt Parfait	Rosemary-Spiced Nuts	Quinoa & Black Bean Salad Jars	Grilled Peach with Ricotta and Basil	Slow-Cooked Mediterranean Chicken
Day 11	Savory Muffin Tin Omelettes	Chilled Cucumber Cups	Chicken and Walnut Pesto Wraps	Blueberry Mango Chia Pudding	Tuscan Pork Tenderloin
Day 12	Smoked Salmon and Herb Cream Cheese Wraps	Smoked Salmon & Cream Cheese Pinwheels	Mediterranean Tuna and Barley Salad	Strawberry Rhubarb Compote with Mint	One-Pan Salmon with Asparagus
Day 13	Chia and Coconut Yogurt Parfait	Cauliflower Tabbouleh	Sardine and Chickpea Salad Pita	Grilled Peach with Ricotta and Basil	Zucchini Ribbon Salad with Lemon and Herbs
Day 14	Chia and Almond Yogurt Parfait	Cucumber Roll-Ups with Feta and Sun-dried Tomatoes	Spicy Pumpkin Soup	Almond Butter Chocolate Energy Balls	Zucchini Ribbon and Turkey Bacon Skillet
Day 15	Peaches and Cream Oat Shake	Chilled Cucumber Cups	Quinoa & Black Bean Salad Jars	Almond Flour Lemon Cake	Slow-Cooked Mediterranean Chicken

	breakfast	snack	lunch	snack	dinner
Day 16	Smoked Salmon and Avocado Tartine	Smoked Salmon & Cream Cheese Pinwheels	Smoked Chicken Caesar Lettuce Wrap	Pumpkin Spice Muffins with Stevia	Lemon Herb Roasted Chicken Thighs
Day 17	Berry Ginger Zinger Smoothie	Herbed Ricotta and Chive Spread	Seared Tuna and Avocado Salad	Coconut Chia Pudding	Tuscan Pork Tenderloin
Day 18	Spinach and Mushroom Egg Muffins	Spicy Bok Choy in Garlic Sauce	Beetroot and Goat Cheese Arugula Salad	Spiced Baked Pear Halves	Zesty Lemon Garlic Tilapia
Day 19	Cucumber Melon Medley Shake	Roasted Red Pepper and Walnut Dip	Tempeh and Kale Pesto Wrap	Almond Flour Lemon Bars	Spiced Cauliflower Steaks with Turmeric and Cumin
Day 20	Turmeric Tofu Scramble	Zucchini Basil Bites	Tomato Basil Soup	Blueberry Mango Chia Pudding	One-Pan Salmon with Asparagus
Day 21	Broccoli and Feta Omelet	Rosemary-Spiced Nuts	Broccoli and Cheddar Soup	No-Bake Lemon Cheesecake Cups	Cauliflower Steaks with Romesco Sauce
Day 22	Chia and Hemp Seed Yogurt Parfait	Spicy Pumpkin Seed Dip	Cucumber and Fennel Citrus Salad	Pistachio and Date Bars	Stuffed Bell Peppers with Quinoa and Turkey
Day 23	Smoked Salmon and Herb Cream Cheese Wraps	Roasted Chickpea and Kale Poppers	Chicken and Walnut Pesto Wraps	Coconut Flour Chocolate Chip Cookies	Herb Crusted Salmon with Fennel Salad
Day 24	Savory Muffin Tin Omelettes	Roasted Acorn Squash with Herbs and Pecans	Mediterranean Tuna and Barley Salad	Strawberry Rhubarb Compote with Mint	Grilled Tofu and Asparagus with Tahini Sauce
Day 25	Peaches and Cream Oat Shake	Spicy Pumpkin Seed Dip	Tempeh and Kale Pesto Wrap	Pistachio and Date Bars	Zucchini Ribbon Salad with Lemon and Herbs
Day 26	Berry Ginger Zinger Smoothie	Roasted Acorn Squash with Herbs and Pecans	Tomato Basil Soup	Pumpkin Spice Muffins with Stevia	One-Pan Salmon with Asparagus
Day 27	Smoked Salmon and Avocado Tartine	Smoked Salmon & Cream Cheese Pinwheels	Spicy Pumpkin Soup	Spiced Baked Pear Halves	Herb Crusted Salmon with Fennel Salad
Day 28	Savory Muffin Tin Omelettes	Rosemary-Spiced Nuts	Seared Tuna and Avocado Salad	Blueberry Mango Chia Pudding	Spiced Cauliflower Steaks with Turmeric and Cumin
Day 29	Cucumber Melon Medley Shake	Zucchini Basil Bites	Broccoli and Cheddar Soup	No-Bake Lemon Cheesecake Cups	Slow-Cooked Mediterranean Chicken
Day 30	Chia and Almond Yogurt Parfait	Chilled Cucumber Cups	Sardine and Chickpea Salad Pita	Coconut Chia Pudding	Stuffed Bell Peppers with Quinoa and Turkey

Conclusion

As we close this culinary journey, I invite you to pause for a moment and marvel at the path we've traversed together through the pages of this cookbook. It's not just a compilation of recipes; it's a testament to the possibilities that embrace us when we choose to confront our health challenges head-on, especially diabetes after the age of 50. It's about transforming limitations into opportunities, turning every meal into a celebration of life, health, and wellbeing.

Managing diabetes in the later stages of life comes with its complexities. You might have noticed over the past chapters how prioritizing a low-carb and low-sugar diet is akin to learning a new language—the language of your body. Speaking this language fluently allows you to understand more deeply what your body needs and how it reacts to different foods. By now, it's quite likely that words like "glycemic index," "whole foods," and "nutrient density" have become part of your everyday vocabulary. Through our recipes and meal plans, we've seen how these concepts materialize into delicious, nourishing meals.

Consider the journey of Mark, a 55-year-old who recently faced the daunting diagnosis of type 2 diabetes. Like many, he felt overwhelmed. His love for cooking was tinged with fear—fear that his kitchen, once a place of joy, was now a minefield of restrictions. However, Mark's story changed when he began seeing his diet as a canvas rather than a cage. With each recipe in this book, he transformed his fear into creativity, understanding that each ingredient he chose was a building block to better health. Mark is not a figment of imagination but a composite of many who have walked this path, finding solace and success in their new dietary lifestyle.

This shift—from fear to empowerment—is what I hope for you. Every example in this book, every tip about managing carb intake or choosing the right fats, is designed to fortify this transformation.

Hand in hand with learning the ropes of this new diet comes an emotional journey. It's perfectly normal to occasionally feel deprived or even frustrated. Social gatherings might seem daunting as you navigate a buffet of potential spikes in blood sugar. Here, the key is planning and confidence—confidence in your ability to make choices that align with your health goals. Remember, every small victory counts. Every time you choose a low-carb appetizer or a sugar-free drink, you're reinforcing your commitment to your health.

Now, I'd like to address a crucial element that extends beyond the dinner plate: the emotional sustenance derived from community. Sharing your experiences, whether challenges in adapting recipes or the joy of discovering a new favorite meal, can immensely boost your motivation. Engaging with support groups, whether online or in your local community, serves as a reminder that you are not navigating this path alone. In these communities, shared experiences act as both a mirror and a window—they reflect your journey and provide a vista of new possibilities.

Furthermore, let us not forget the influence of regular physical activity and its role in managing diabetes. A walk around the neighborhood or gentle yoga can complement your dietary efforts, helping in managing your blood sugar levels and enhancing your overall sense of wellbeing.

Looking ahead, I encourage you to view this book not just as a reference but as a companion. As seasons change, so may your dietary needs and preferences. Use what you've learned here to adapt, to continue experimenting with flavors and textures while keeping your health in focus. Whether it's tweaking recipes to celebrate the holidays, experimenting with new vegetarian dishes, or mastering the grill for a summer cookout, each occasion is an opportunity to reaffirm your commitment to a healthier, happier you.

Lastly, I urge you to carry forward the optimism that has been a thread throughout this book. The journey with diabetes is ongoing and evolving. New research might open up additional pathways for managing your condition, and staying informed is key. Always consult with healthcare providers to tailor any general advice to your specific health conditions.

Remember, managing diabetes effectively does not mean relinquishing joy in what you eat. It's about creating a balanced, delightful diet that supports your health and satisfies your soul. It's about redefining boundaries, not being confined by them. As you continue on this path, remember that each meal is more than just food on a plate—it's an affirmation of your life and your health. Here's to a future where every bite is tasty, and every day is a step towards lasting wellness. Thank you for allowing this book to be a part of your journey.

MEASUREMENT CONVERSION TABLE

Volume Measurements

US Measurement	Metric Measurement
1 tsp (tsp)	5 milliliters (ml)
1 tbsp (tbsp)	15 milliliters (ml)
1 fluid ounce (fl oz)	30 milliliters (ml)
1 Cup	240 milliliters (ml)
1 pint (2 Cs)	470 milliliters (ml)
1 quart (4 Cs)	0.95 liters (L)
1 gallon (16 Cs)	3.8 liters (L)

Weight Measurements

US Measurement	Metric Measurement
1 ounce (oz)	28 grams (g)
1 pound (lb)	450 grams (g)
1 pound (lb)	0.45 kilograms (kg)

Length Measurements

US Measurement	Metric Measurement
1 inch (in)	2.54 centimeters (cm)
1 foot (ft)	30.48 centimeters (cm)
1 foot (ft)	0.3048 meters (m)
1 yard (yd)	0.9144 meters (m)

Temperature Conversions

Fahrenheit (°F)	Celsius (°C)
32°F	0°C
212°F	100°C
Formula: (°F - 32) x 0.5556 = °C	Formula: (°C x 1.8) + 32 = °F

Oven Temperature Conversions

US Oven Term	Fahrenheit (°F)	Celsius (°C)
Very Slow	250°F	120°C
Slow	300-325°F	150-165°C
Moderate	350-375°F	175-190°C
Moderately Hot	400°F	200°C
Hot	425-450°F	220-230°C
Very Hot	475-500°F	245-260°C

Made in the USA
Columbia, SC
06 January 2025